THE **WEIGHT LOSS PLAN** FOR
BEATING
DIABETES

THE **WEIGHT LOSS PLAN** FOR
BEATING
DIABETES

The **5-Step Program** That Removes Metabolic Roadblocks,
Sheds Pounds Safely, and Reverses Prediabetes and Diabetes

FREDERIC J. VAGNINI, M.D., FACS
AND **LAWRENCE D. CHILNICK**

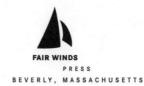

FAIR WINDS
PRESS
BEVERLY, MASSACHUSETTS

Text © 2009 Frederic J. Vagnini, M.D., FACS, and Lawrence D. Chilnick

First published in the USA in 2009 by
Fair Winds Press, a member of
Quayside Publishing Group
100 Cummings Center
Suite 406-L
Beverly, MA 01915-6101
www.fairwindspress.com

13 12 11 10 09   1 2 3 4 5

ISBN-13: 978-1-59233-384-4
ISBN-10: 1-59233-384-2

Library of Congress Cataloging-in-Publication Data

Cover design by Andrew Brozyna
Book design by Colleen Cunningham

Printed and bound in Canada

The information in this book is for educational purposes only. It is not intended
to replace the advice of a physician or medical practitioner. Please see your
health-care provider before beginning any new health program.

This book is dedicated to Susan Hill, R.N., a loyal friend of over thirty years. Susan has been the director of my cardiac, vascular, and metabolic services at my centers for over thirty years. She has been an integral part in managing the thousands of patients that have been treated for heart, vascular, and metabolic problems. Without her, much of what I have accomplished would not have been possible. I deeply appreciate, beyond her imagination, the dedication, work professionalism, friendship, and commitment of Susan.

Frederic J. Vagnini, M.D., FACS

To the continued health of the "Chilnicks": Susanna, Jeremy, Janet, Judy, and EJ for their care, support and love helping me regain my own health and "being there" always.

Lawrence D. Chilnick

CONTENTS

PART TWO: LIVING AND LOSING WEIGHT IN THE REAL WORLD

Foreword

In our many years of research and teaching at Mt. Sinai School of Medicine and in the City University of New York, and in our personal lives as well, we have often been asked how best to judge medical advice.

"How do I know what to do?" a newly diagnosed diabetic may ask. "One book says one thing, another book says another. Then you listen to the six o'clock news and you hear something completely different!"

It's true. In this wide world of instant communication and free speech, anyone can claim to be an expert and anyone's advice may be right on target ... or may be dead wrong.

We have found there are three simple three rules that work best in determining the value of health-related advice: First, consider the source. Second and third, consider the source.

The value of the advice is only as good as the person giving it.

With that standard in mind, it is with pure pleasure that we write the foreword to this book.

We have had the pleasure of knowing Dr. Frederic Vagnini for over two decades. We have spent untold hours discussing the latest research in heart disease, weight loss, and diabetes. In person, on the phone, or by e-mail, our communications are almost always part-personal and part-biomedical science. For Dr. V., as he is affectionately called by his myriad patients, scientific knowledge is not something a physician should seek when it is needed. For this respected physician, scientific knowledge it is a precious commodity to be accumulated and stored away for the patient whose life might well be affected or saved by it.

We were brought together by Dr. V.'s personal quest to lose weight. He was warm and easygoing. We were soon to learn, however, that beneath that likable exterior lay a razor-sharp mind and an uncompromising commitment to his own health and weight loss.

In the twenty years that have followed, we have seen Dr. V. bring that same set of admirable qualities to the care of both his patients and his readers. In our opinion, no other author could bring a greater knowledge, understanding, or personal commitment to a book on diabetes and weight loss.

One final, personal note: Although our knowledge of the health-related issues and treatments is vast, before we make an important health-related decision for ourselves, we typically conclude: "We'd better call Fred."

—Rachel F. Heller, M.A., M.Ph., Ph.D. and Richard Heller, M.S., Ph.D.

Introduction: My Story

People who have read my previous books know that I suffered through obesity and poor health issues myself. But how did it all start? How did a young man who had always been in good physical condition turn into someone with obesity, severe health problems, prediabetes, and lipid abnormalities? The fact is that my struggle with weight is not that different from yours. I am a walking example of a person who has taken charge of his bad health habits and turned things around. Here's a little of my story.

Growing up in an Italian family, life was all about food, family, and family gatherings. Three things were important: food, food, and food all of the time—and much of it "bad for you" food.

I remember my associations with food well when I think about my childhood in Astoria, Queens. Breakfast was a carbohydrate delight, featuring Wheaties with sugar, bananas, milk, and orange juice. Each day I walked to public school 126, which was two blocks away from my family's home on Crescent Street. Because it was just a short walk, I came home for lunch, and my mother always had some type of sandwich and tomato soup with rice (note the carbs and sugar). And every day she gave me 10 cents to buy a large pretzel on my way back to school. The pretzels were soft, fresh, and chewy, a carbohydrate addict's delight, and I think they started my carbohydrate addiction.

Just growing up in Astoria was another problem because we walked past La Guli Italian pastries every Sunday on our way to church. A few blocks away was the famous Walken's bakery. Right at the base of the elevated train station on Broadway was a *Parisi* Italian bread store, and of course you had to get a couple of loaves of bread when you went by because the mere smell of it made you hungry.

Food Addictions Begin to Take Hold

When I was young, I also had my own special food addictions such as Twinkies. These provoked a sort of Pavlovian response just thinking about them as I did every night when my sisters, Grace and Ann, and I were growing up. Often, too, around nine at night, my father would give us a dollar to go to Jenny's Grocery Store around the corner to get a quart of hand-packed ice cream. This became another addictive problem.

When I was in grammar school and high school, sometimes as a snack, Mom would prepare white bread with sugar on it. That does not seem to be such a great idea now.

Mom's amazing cooking didn't help. One of her specialties, especially around the holidays, was pantaloons. These ravioli-like treats were prepared with chocolate chickpea dough, with a chickpea filling drenched with honey, quite a sugar overload as I think about it now. Mom was also famous for her chocolate cake, which we called "cockroach cake" because it had pignoli nuts in it, and their color for some reason prompted that nasty name. Despite its name, it tasted great, and it too was addicting.

Here's another example of Mom's cooking style: My mother fried her famous meatballs in Crisco and served them to the family and neighbors every Sunday through the window in front of our summer house in Bayville, Long Island.

Delicious everyday meals were the rule, filled with pasta, meatballs, and delicious bread. Every day at my house was kind of a feast. In later years, when I brought college friends over, suddenly a full meal complete with desserts would appear. My mother always had pies and cakes and many other specialty items on hand.

Growing up, we also had a summer house in Bayville, New York, and there my Uncle Leo took over. (As you might guess by now, my entire family had no problem with food. Many were obese, and looking back at their pictures now,

I am sure they were also diabetic. Two of my uncles died in their fifties.) Uncle Leo's barbeques were also great, with hot dogs and hamburgers, lots of fresh sweet corn (more carbohydrates), and a lovely soda fountain that dispensed high sugar, grape syrup drink to all the kids. At night at Uncle Leo's, we had a watermelon club, where basically all my cousins, family, and my Uncle Leo ate a 50-pound (22.7 kg) watermelon every week during the summer—more sugar and more carbohydrates.

It was all such an addicting process through the years that it was amazing that I maintained my thin body build through college, medical school, and my internship and residency.

Then It All Caught Up to Me

How did it happen? It seemed to occur overnight, but the start of it was in one of my offices, when a physician friend came in and said, "Doc, you have high cholesterol."

I replied, "You're crazy, my cholesterol is fine. And how would you know? I haven't even had a blood test!"

He was right. I had a condition called "xanthalesma," which are fatty yellow deposits of cholesterol around the eyes and eyelids, which I never realized I had.

I did a blood study, and I had high cholesterol and also high triglycerides. I was not even heavy at that time. I started myself on lipid-lowering therapy, and almost immediately I gained weight rather than lost it. After some health problems and some personal tragedies, I weighed 325 pounds (147.4 kg).

My clothes no longer fit, and I didn't have any answers. I didn't know what to do. I could only wear one of my sports jackets. Yet hanging in my closet was an entire wardrobe of custom-made suits, which I no longer fit into.

One day I looked in the mirror with my shirt off and realized that I was fat! I said to myself, I cannot believe it, this is not me. But it was, and I really got the message when I had to go out one day to buy "fat man" clothes. I returned in a baggy leisure suit, got in front of the mirror, and was brought to tears because it was obvious that I had become obese.

I also had no energy. The turning point was one day when I was lying on the couch, my two daughters Grace and Clare at my side. I was always exhausted after eating, and I asked myself, How can I take care of these children? I won't be here for them if they need me in an emergency. I don't think I can even get off the couch. I can still recall pushing my daughter's stroller up a slight hill one day. I couldn't make it, so I had to sit down on the curb.

Time to Change

My weight problem was really getting to me. I can even recall taking two sandwiches to bed at night, one to have watching the late show and the other during the middle of the night, when I probably had severe hypoglycemia. It was a crazy time because I also smoked then. I drank alcohol, too, probably in excess.

I finally started to study dieting. I got some bad information at first, from a nutritionist who worked in my office telling me pasta is good. When I got deeper into the subject of diet and nutrition, which was not usual for me since I was a cardiovascular surgeon, I found people had been successful with the Scarsdale-type of diet, which is a low carbohydrate diet.

I started on that program, but was still struggling until fortunately one of my patients introduced me to the concept of carbohydrate addictions. I interviewed Rachel F. Heller, M.A., M.Ph., Ph.D., and Richard Heller, M.S., Ph.D., authors and advocates of this approach, who have subsequently become very close friends, colleagues, and a mini-support group. With the help of Rachel and Richard and their dietary program, I turned myself around. I lost more than 100 pounds (45.4 kg), and got myself down to about 200 pounds (90.7 kg), which was almost too thin.

I never really exercised when losing the weight, I didn't really feel well enough to, but when I lost most of my muscle mass, I realized I had to start exercising. I began with a treadmill and went on to resistance training and weight training, which has been very important in maintaining my health. As I went through the process, I also learned about nutraceuticals (which are extracts of foods, plants, or other natural substances that many scientists and physicians believe have a positive effect on health and healing) and lifestyle changes, as you will later in the book. Today, many years later, I still have a relatively good body build with a lean body mass. Although I remain predia-betic, my lipids and my blood pressure are satisfactory, and my hormonal markers, which measure any negative chemical activity such as reduced insulin levels, are in good balance.

PART ONE: THE FIVE ESSENTIAL STEPS TO DIABETIC WEIGHT LOSS

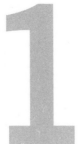

Discover Why This Program Is for You

You should know three things about diabetes, obesity, and weight loss. First, your weight problem as a diabetic is likely *not your fault*. Second, the program in this book *costs you nothing*, and it is not a "product" of a prepackaged diet industry, where many of the diets or products have a 90 percent failure rate. Third, the reason you can't seem to lose weight and keep it off is that you have a series of metabolic roadblocks, but they can be surmounted whether you have prediabetes or type 2 diabetes.

Oh, one more thing: You are not alone. Millions of people are fighting the same weight loss battle you are. More people around the world die from obesity than starvation: One billion are obese or overweight compared with 800 million who are underweight. According to the World Health Organization, "Overweight and obese people outnumber the undernourished in the world, and childhood obesity is now so widespread that for the first time in history, the human race is facing the possibility of millions of parents outliving their children."

The obesity epidemic in the United States is one of the reasons the incidence of diabetes has doubled in the past decade. And the incidence, according to the

Centers for Disease Control and Prevention (CDC), is highest in the states where obesity is highest.

This information is not news. It has been widely discussed for years, and it was first published in medical journals in 2006. My own patient treatment programs and research and my colleagues' studies now indisputably confirm something that's been obvious for years: Obesity—even just being overweight—makes you a prime candidate for diabetes and heart disease, and without *serious intervention* you'll probably end up taking multiple medications and/or having to make drastic lifestyle alterations for a disease that can affect your work, sex life, and vision, and even cause premature death. Other problems often seen in obese people with diabetes are Alzheimer's disease and dementia. Do you want to prevent all of these life-shortening, cardio-metabolic risks, avoid potentially catastrophic illness, and live a longer and healthier life? Then this book and the weight loss plan within it will help save you.

LEARN ABOUT THE UNIQUE FEATURES OF THE PLAN

Why, though, do you need another weight loss book? After all, most brand-name plans begin by making an outlandish promise of weight loss through a "breakthrough" that somehow the hundreds of other programs missed.

The answer is simple: This book's weight loss program is designed specifically to help people with diabetes and the 57 million people in the United States—more than 40 percent of adults according to the CDC—who are in a temporary "safety zone," which is called "prediabetes." One reason this plan works is because it tells you how to remove *all* of the metabolic roadblocks that diabetes creates. This method of treating diabetes and prediabetes literally creates weight loss through a sort of biological chain reaction as you become healthier through proper diabetic treatment.

Studies show that even if your loss is not significant, perhaps only 5 to 7 percent of your body weight, you can reduce the chances of progressing from impaired glucose tolerance (IGT) to type 2 diabetes by 58 percent.

Even if you gain the weight back, you will have helped your diabetes. Studies at Kaiser Permanente Northwest in Portland, Oregon, report that the therapeutic benefits achieved by losing weight are sustained, even if the patients eventually regain the weight.

The Five-Step Plan in this book also considers something that you would think is an obvious and bottom-line criterion in any weight loss program: It takes into account the fact that no two people are the same. (Virtually no other weight loss plan does this.) This is an important fact, especially for people with diabetes. For example, someone with diabetes might have cardio-vascular disease, increased heart attack risk, vision loss, high blood pressure, lipid abnormalities, increased atherosclerotic process, and is markedly more at risk for stroke, Alzheimer's disease, and cancer. All of these, coupled with diabetes itself, as you will see in this book, affect weight gain and loss.

Even in people with a family history of diabetes, their risk factor for diabetes can affect them in myriad ways. This is why there are so many "shades" of the disease, which makes losing weight a person-specific task.

The other facet of this book that sets it apart from other weight loss books is that overcoming denial and noncompliance with medical treatments are also part of this weight loss program. These self-imposed weight loss obstacles that you as a prediabetic or diabetic face are similar to a broken red light that never changes to green. If you don't fix it, you will remain where you are, and your personal health problems will continue to build up—like traffic.

LOSE WEIGHT—AT LAST

In all my years of medical practice, not one patient has said, "Dr. Vagnini, I'd like to eat until I explode." Or "I'd like to be so overweight that I have to buy two seats on the airplane." There is no question that you, especially as diabetic, do not want to be overweight or obese. Virtually everyone seeking to lose weight has gone through what is often called weight cycling—losses and gains. This is not necessarily a negative because it indicates that you are still trying. There is little hard data on this subject, but some experts say that the average person who diets goes through at least ten different diets or weight loss programs in a lifetime. Like any activity, learning to play tennis or learning to drive, it might take some time for all of the pieces to fall into place. Controlling your diabetes to achieve permanent weight loss is also a learning process that you have to dedicate yourself to mastering.

This is one promise of this book to you, but there are many more. You *can* be helped because weight gain as a diabetic is not your fault, and everything contributing to it can be reversed. Losing weight as a diabetic can be a long-term process because the disease itself builds slowly, which is one of the reasons that doctors use the catchall term *pre*diabetes.

The complications of diabetes—the nerve, artery, heart, and vascular damage—take years and years to develop. We do know that with the right help—the right motivation and the right program—the weight problems and medical problems can be turned around so that you can lead a normal, healthy life.

"I frequently tell people when I see them in the office, as I told a young man who was in recently (he was in his mid-forties, but he looked like a teenager), I say, 'I'm not treating you for today; I'm treating you twenty years from now because you know how the sands go through the hourglass. It's grain by grain, and before you realize it's all gone and you're in trouble.'"

SAVE MONEY BY LOSING WEIGHT

Many sociological side effects of diabetes and obesity often go unnoticed. The economic burden of this disease on this country is staggering. Studies conducted a decade ago showed that the costs were over $20 billion a year, 50 percent of which was for treatment alone. Today, according to new pharmaceutical industry studies, the costs are now well over $200 billion! This includes all the direct medical expenses from visits to the doctor to medication and hospitalizations, plus loss of productivity on the part of the patients.

strange but true

Oddly enough, despite the diagnosis of more than 1.6 million new cases a year in the United States, diabetes is not feared as it should be. A survey taken by the ADA and the CDC and published in *Diabetes in Control,* showed that the respondents were more afraid of "shark bites, plane crashes, or cancer. These fears exist despite the fact that there were only 70 confirmed shark bites and 491 deaths in plane crashes in 2007. There were 233,429 deaths related directly to diabetes."

Think about this in another way: Diabetes costs are now 10 percent of the entire U.S. health-care budget, and diabetes is responsible for 50 percent of the costs of heart disease and stroke combined.

These are costs for a disease that is highly preventable and whose treatments can be reduced through a wellness approach to health.

It does not have to be this way: Weight loss in a diabetic can cut health-care costs directly.

According to the American Diabetes Association (ADA), "Data gathered from an HMO claims database (1997–2005) showed that study participants with diabetes who experienced 1 percent weight loss decreased their average health-care costs by 3.6 percent over the 12 months following the weight loss, or approximately $256. Results were even more significant among patients considered obese (BMI [body mass index] greater than or equal to 30). For this group, a 1 percent weight loss was associated with a 5.6 percent decrease in health care costs, or approximately $408."

diabetes and obesity facts

- According to the World Health Organization and the Centers for Disease Control and Prevention there are about 1 billion overweight people in the world, of whom 400 million are obese; if this is an accurate figure, it equates to a world epidemic.

- Obesity is now the greatest contributor to chronic disease.

- Obesity increases the risk of progression to permanent atrial fibrillation (abnormal heart rhythm).

- Young women between eighteen and thirty-five are gaining weight more quickly than any other age group. This is a concern because as many as 50 percent of women who are obese develop type 2 diabetes within five years. Experts say young women are in denial about the medical risks of being overweight.

- Obesity among young women has been blamed for quadrupling the number of pregnant women with gestational diabetes. This condition increases the risk of pregnancy complications, such as having a larger baby, which makes labor and delivery harder.

- In 2007, at least 57 million Americans had prediabetes.

- More than 20 million adults, adolescents, and children have diabetes. The American Diabetes Association estimates that an additional 6 million people are not even aware of their risk for the disease or that they already have it.

BUST SOME DIABETES MYTHS

Let's start by removing one of the most important roadblocks to losing weight with diabetes—myths and misunderstanding about diabetes. Health care is filled with myths, and diabetes, which causes considerable heart, blood pressure, and nerve damage, vision and weight problems, is a leading source of those myths. At the root of many of these misunderstandings is word-of-mouth opinion spread from one patient to another like a virulent infection. Add to that confusing and conflicting media reports about medication and the validity of treatments that are popular in one place and disavowed in others. Even "official" organizations add to the confusion by releasing statements that significantly redefine the guidelines your doctor has been using to determine whether you have prediabetes or type 2 diabetes.

So, if you take seriously what you hear from your relatives in Florida who are quoting their neighbors or their cousin's son—the dermatologist—you are placing yourself at risk.

Let's take a look at a few of the myths that may be holding you back. The following self test will give you an idea of what you think is true or false about certain aspects of both weight loss and type 2 diabetes. Circle "true" or "false" for each statement below.

1. Diabetes is contagious.   True   False
2. If you have diabetes, you'll never be able to eat a chocolate
    bar again.   True   False
3. People with diabetes have to eat special food.   True   False
4. Pasta is a thing of the past for people with diabetes.   True   False
5. People with diabetes are frequently sick.   True   False
6. Sugar causes diabetes.   True   False
7. Insulin is dangerous and makes you fat.   True   False
8. People with diabetes can eat as much fruit as they want.   True   False
9. An A1C of 8 means your diabetes is okay.   True   False
10. Only certain kinds of diabetes are serious.   True   False
11. None of my siblings have diabetes so I won't develop it.   True   False
12. Once you take medication, you can live any way you want.   True   False
13. People with diabetes usually have erectile dysfunction.   True   False
14. Type 2 diabetes is less serious than type 1.   True   False
15. Everyone has a blood sugar level that is okay for them.   True   False

16. Exercise can cure diabetes.	True	False
17. Losing weight will also cure diabetes.	True	False
18. Vitamins and supplements are a waste of money for people with diabetes.	True	False
19. People with diabetes should eat bananas for potassium.	True	False
20. Controlling your diabetes ensures that you won't have a heart attack.	True	False
21. You can cure diabetes and never have it again.	True	False

What were your answers? How many did you mark as "true" or "false"?

Here's the surprise. Every one of these twenty-one statements is *false*! Physicians hear these common myths all the time.

As you proceed, you'll find out why these myths are so widely thought to be true. As you come to understand why they are myths, your knowledge will increase and your weight loss and diabetes control efforts will begin to pay off.

What you will also come to understand in this book is why you need a five-step plan that begins with education and adds medication and natural supplements to a way of eating that millions of healthy people around the world already follow. That's why this book is focused on two things:

1. Weight loss
2. Control of your prediabetes or type 2 diabetes

You will learn how to achieve these two things over the rest of this book, and equally important, it will dispel the myths and misunderstandings that accompany chronic illness such as type 2 diabetes. The chapters that follow will hand you the keys to the destruction of both biological and psychological roadblocks you may have created to prevent weight loss.

THE MORE YOU KNOW ABOUT YOUR ROADBLOCKS, THE MORE YOU CAN LOSE

There are two basic reasons why so many people who have prediabetes have lost control of their weight and are teetering on the cusp of obesity. First, you may not know that you are at risk, so your weight gain, poor diet, and lifestyle may lead to full-fledged type 2 diabetes. Then once you have diabetes, you may not realize that losing weight is a different challenge than it is for every other person and every other diabetic.

Someone with diabetes who needs to lose weight must recognize it's simply not going to happen with a fad or branded diet because diabetic obesity is a result of a set of roadblocks—metabolic disorders—that have to be treated properly. The reason that the plan in this book works is you will learn how to target these roadblocks and overcome them. Defeating, treating, and reducing these roadblocks is an approach to diabetic weight loss that you will not find anywhere else. This is why prepackaged, microwave dinners usually won't work, especially over the long run, for someone with diabetes who must lose weight.

Step One of our Five-Step Plan, learning all you can about the biological roots and causes of your prediabetes or diabetes, is an obvious starting point.

Knowledge gives you greater ability to control your condition and to attack the metabolic roadblocks that diabetes has created. Facts will give you power and the fortitude you need because losing weight and keeping it off, especially when you have diabetes, is a significant challenge. You must recognize just how much your ability to understand the different, targeted medical treatments and to make wise choices about complying with those treatments is linked to losing weight and prolonging your life.

People with prediabetes and diabetes *will* lose weight through this plan's combination of activities and treatments. I've put them into a five-step program because one step builds upon the previous step to help you maintain health and to provide benchmarks to keep you motivated. Thousands of people with diabetes have successfully used this system, which was developed over fifteen years ago at the Heart, Diabetes and Weight Loss Center of New York.

Step One of the Five-Step Plan begins with education (I like to call it an information injection) because knowledge is the foundation for any task. Information is even more important to weight loss. As you read and absorb the basics about diabetes weight loss in this section, keep in mind that this is only the first part of the plan. You can only ensure success by following up with Steps Two through Five, including:

- Which medications work in combination with others
- Building an eating plan with your unique health issues and complications in mind
- Which supplements ("nutraceuticals") can aid the cause
- Proper exercise
- Lifestyle changes that complete the picture

IDENTIFY CHALLENGES

As a diabetic on a weight loss program, your path is similar to a person traveling a road filled with fallen trees and boulders. Physiological, sociological, and genetic roadblocks abound. These challenges occur everywhere. Some are built-in; others you will encounter in the supermarket while planning a family dinner, when remembering to take medication properly, and when trying to maintain a healthful lifestyle while at work or traveling. Many of these road-blocks are not identified until you have a complete medical workup as described later in this chapter, so it's important to understand them as soon as you can and this is why they are up front in the education step.

Here is a rundown of these roadblocks. How you respond to them with the help of this book will determine your ultimate ability to lose weight and lessen the severity of your diabetes.

Metabolic syndrome: Lifestyle and "food-style" factors lead to this number one problem that people with diabetes face in losing weight. If you have the following cluster of conditions right now, you likely have it.

- Visceral adiposity: the belly fat, or roll of fat around the waist, that we all fight to eliminate is one of the most important diabetic roadblocks
- High blood pressure
- Low HDL cholesterol ("good cholesterol")
- High triglycerides
- Elevated blood glucose levels—also known as hyperglycemia—causing too much insulin to enter your system and damage your organs

Inability to burn fat because of metabolic changes, such as elevated triglycerides. The presence of visceral fat signals a lack of fat breakdown and elevated blood glucose.

Genetics: It's hard to escape genetics. As explained later, knowing your family history of diabetes and sharing this information with your doctor is critical. Your genetic risk essentially makes you more likely than the rest of the population to become diabetic if you place yourself in jeopardy through poor diet or lack of exercise. Knowing your genetic background should alert your physician to counsel you and to recommend regular checkups and blood tests.

Ethnic heritage: Your ethnic heritage is also part of your genetic makeup. Many of us are raised in ethnic cultures with diets loaded with filling foods and carbohydrates. Culturally driven behavior is an important roadblock to weight loss. This is especially true in cultural groups such as Italians, which led me to become addicted to bread and pasta. Latino or Hispanic diets, too, feature high carbohydrates such as rice and beans, and geographic regions such as the U.S. South are known for things such as heavy fried foods. While some of this may seem stereotypical, it is actually quite common. In Step Three, you will learn how to overcome this problem.

Fluctuating insulin and glucose levels: This is perhaps the toughest roadblock for most people with diabetes, especially those who also are obese. This fluctuation creates a yo-yo effect as your glucose level drops and you become hungry. If you eat too many carbs to bring it up, you will gain weight. This pattern leads to cravings, bingeing, and uncontrolled eating.

Stress: Emotional stress leads to emotional eating, which is complicated by the increased release of the hormones cortisol and catecholamine, that raise dopamine, norepinephrine, and epinephrine levels. This process is associated with weight increase in diabetics, and it also can lead to heart disease, hypertension, reduced immune function, and fatal diseases such as cancer as well as an alteration in blood glucose levels resulting in hunger, bingeing and craving, and increased fat storage.

Brain fog: This is a secondary development from high glucose levels caused by reduced blood flow to the brain cells: The person is "out of it." Reduced blood flow causes patients to ignore what they are told, and they don't help themselves. It also results in fatigue, loss of motivation, and inactivity.

Fatigue: Overweight people with diabetes are often fatigued, and it is related to hormone decline (especially testosterone in men) and diminished thyroid and adrenal function and adrenal fatigue. It becomes impossible to exercise, which is an important part of the weight loss program. Fatigue in turn adds to depression.

Nonalcoholic steatohepatitis hepatitis (NASH): There is a frequent incidence of NASH among certain people with type 2 diabetes that affects the liver. People with this condition appear to have liver disease, but they may not have any symptoms and do not necessarily drink significant amounts of alcohol. NASH patients that have fatty livers are less able to detoxify their bodies, leaving them more prone to fatigue and with an overall feeling of malaise.

Musculoskeletal problems: It's not uncommon to see obese patients, with or without diabetes, who have severe knee and lower back problems. Their weight increases degenerative bone and muscle disease, leading to the inability to exercise or even walk as a result of stiffness, joint pain, and progressive joint disease. There is an increased incidence of arthritis in obese diabetics.

Postprandial hyperglycemia: This is a rise in blood sugar after a meal, possibly from eating too many carbohydrates. When that happens, you get sleepy, which, in turn, leads to less thermogenesis, the normal bodily function that generates heat and energy. Although your metabolism is stoked with energy-producing fuel, the energy isn't being burned by physical activity, so you gain weight, which leads to an inability to exercise, leading to failure to burn calories, leading to—well, you get the picture. A similar situation occurs with late night eating.

Gastroenterological problems: In people with diabetes, these may include gastroesophageal reflux disease (GERD), hypochlorhydria (a lack of, or too little, stomach acid that in turn hinders digestion), and gastritis, which may be caused by taking too many h2 blockers such as ranitidine (brand name Zantac), nizatidine (brand name Axid), cimetidine (brand name Tagamet), or famotidine (brand name Pepcid) to treat indigestion. Chronic constipation and irritable bowel syndrome might also accompany poor eating habits and a toxic lifestyle.

Dysbiosis: This is the presence of abnormal bacterial flora in the gut and is common in overweight diabetics. It can lead to food allergies; altered gut permeability (i.e., the inability to absorb food and excrete waste materials into the intestines); and fatigue, gas, and bloating.

Candidasis: This occurs frequently in overweight people with diabetes as a result of an overgrowth of *Candida albicans*, a form of yeast in the gastrointestinal (GI) system. It frequently occurs with the overconsumption of sweets and carbohydrates. GI and systemic conditions can result, such as bloating, gas, indigestion, and irritable bowel, as well as joint pain, headaches, fatigue, skin rashes, and brain fog. These infections often occur in women as vaginal yeast infections, but men can experience them as well since they arise from a GI problem. Yeast infections frequently occur after antibiotic therapy as well.

Carbohydrate addiction: This is characterized by many of the same symptoms as any other addiction, and it's the diabetic's downfall. When glucose levels are unbalanced, a diabetic's first response is to crave junk food—sweets and starchy foods. Carbohydrate addiction is a major roadblock to weight loss, but this book and others, such as *Carbohydrate Addict's Healthy Heart*, provide a program to overcome it.

People on low-carb diets often experience a problem called carbo-drifting (the actual roadblock). Those who are on a carbohydrate restricted diet (especially those who are severely restricted), whether they plateau (are no longer losing weight) or are doing well, may start to increase their carbohydrate intake. This is acceptable if you continue to have good glucose control, weight loss, and stability; however, it can lead to carbohydrate bingeing and a "carb-coma." This is not a full-blown collapse, more like a desperate need to lie down and take a nap after you eat.

Food allergies and sensitivities: People with diabetes and obesity frequently are allergic to dairy and wheat.

Many people with diabetes have a major problem with gluten sensitivity, too. Gluten, a protein found in barley, oats, rye, and wheat, can cause GI problems resulting in disabling fatigue and a multitude of systemic complaints, as well as difficulty in losing weight.

Fluid retention: Retaining fluid is common in many overweight people with prediabetes and diabetes. It might be the result of excessive intake of carbohydrates and excessive calories as well as increase in salt/sodium intake. Fluid retention further impairs the body's natural methods of detoxification, prevents normal enzymatic reaction, and affects bones and joints as well as the liver.

Hidden alcohol: Alcohol intake frequently contributes to development of obesity. You should discuss your intake of alcohol and other fluids with your physician because alcohol is high in calories and frequently is a contributing factor to weight gain. It's important to remember that any caloric intake can cause weight gain. In fact, it's not unusual for overweight people with diabetes to ingest 20 percent of their daily calories from fluids.

Low testosterone: This is extremely common in men, particularly in those who are overweight, especially with visceral adiposity, or who have prediabetes or diabetes. Side effects include depression, fatigue, low metabolism of fat, loss of libido, erectile dysfunction, impaired insulin sensitivity, and loss of muscle mass. This loss of muscle tone and muscle is a major roadblock to starting an exercise program.

Shopping and advertising sabotage: Anyone who goes shopping or is exposed to food advertising knows that this has to be shut out with education so that good choices can be made.

Heavy metal toxicity: In routine tests for mercury, aluminum, lead and arsenic, heavy metals have been found in blood, hair, or urine. Elevated levels of heavy metals affect enzymes in your system, leading to fatigue and joint problems. This in turn contributes to metabolic derangement, further deteriorating the body's already stressed physiologic mechanisms.

Pulmonary complications: People with obesity and diabetes have an increased incidence of asthma. GERD, which is linked to obesity, frequently leads to pulmonary complications.

Cardiovascular complications: These as well as peripheral vascular disease can be debilitating with fatigue, shortness of breath, and inability to exercise or even walk on many occasions. People with diabetes frequently take multiple cardiovascular drug therapies, which have many side effects that may affect their motivation to exercise and eat properly.

Psychological roadblocks: In diabetes, nothing is a single, uncomplicated event. Simply being diagnosed with diabetes can be a significant roadblock to weight loss. When you discover you have prediabetes or diabetes, the diagnosis alone may depress you or prevent you from exercising to lose weight. Extensive research shows that type 2 diabetes can provoke depression and that depression can increase the risk for developing type 2 diabetes. Your blood sugar may rise or fall, creating carbohydrate addiction and exhaustion.

This program, with its emphasis on diabetes education, enables people with prediabetes and diabetes to gain and maintain control of their condition. Unfortunately, many people with diabetes have no real idea why losing weight and keeping it off are so challenging. Now you do.

All of these roadblocks may seem daunting. However, in this book as you learn more about your disease—and yourself—weight loss will become natural.

TAKE THE LEAP

Are you ready to meet the challenges of losing weight with prediabetes or diabetes? You might not think so if you have failed with other poundage reduction programs that measure success by a number on the scale or the size of your belt. You can go to your bookshelf, pantry, and freezer and toss everything you've used in your previous attempts to lose weight. This is the first book that will actually help you lose weight and keep it off.

Forget what you think you know about weight loss. The science and medical developments that helped create this Five-Step Plan for weight loss are based on the successes of thousands of patients who have lost weight because their diabetes has been diagnosed and treated properly for the first time. Their weight loss comes from understanding diabetes as more than a single disorder, a key aspect of weight loss that you will probably understand for the first time when you follow this plan.

Your past efforts also may have been hindered by the considerable number of weight loss roadblocks described above, created by diabetes and your genetic structure. You have less than one in ten chances of successfully losing weight on your own. For someone with prediabetes or diabetes, the Five-Step

Plan is like winning the lottery! You will start to win the battle against weight gain at last, beginning by learning to assess your DNA risk. We cannot emphasize this more: This program is based on controlling the underlying causes of your weight gain—not just eliminating junk food, hitting the gym, or starving yourself.

Jump-starting and succeeding with this plan requires an "I'm ready" mindset, determination, and commitment that will be reinforced as you learn more about your diabetic problems and weight gain.

DON'T WAIT TO GET STARTED

If you've been diagnosed with prediabetes, you must act quickly. By the time your blood glucose sneaks past a certain level, it's too late, and adding medication is the only answer. You might have developed many other medical conditions associated with uncontrolled diabetes. As a diabetic, your risk of death is 50 percent higher than that of nondiabetics of your same age. In addition, while diabetes care and the medications that go with it can be a difficult part of your life, the inconvenience of controlling your diabetes is far better than the risks you'll run without proper medical care.

Admitting that you have to defeat your diabetes roadblocks is difficult, but it's a necessary leap forward for weight loss.

GET AN ACCURATE DIAGNOSIS

Like so many things in life, diabetes is a spectrum. Knowing exactly where you are on the diabetic spectrum is an important part of the education process.

The tests outlined at the end of this chapter will establish this clearly and in detail. Recent research shows that for many people with diabetes, their disease has been undetected for years in spite of multiple visits to the doctor. Why? Most doctors practice acute or reactive medicine, and they only respond to symptoms, such as a cough or pain. Many physicians don't realize or take advantage of the power of preventive medicine, and in their defense you usually only appear at their offices with the flu or an infection.

Unless your chart shows that you have had significant weight loss since your last visit or you have cardiovascular disease, your primary care physician isn't necessarily going to look for diabetes. (Yes, you read that right: unexplained weight *loss*. People with diabetes often lose weight because they develop a condition called protein wasting and extensive loss of body water.) Your office visit ends, and you walk away with a solution to your immediate problem. Because most doctors don't approach medicine holistically, they don't look beyond your cough or headache. It's important that any doctor's visit cover your cardiovascular and diabetic risk. If it doesn't, you're facing another roadblock to good health and weight loss. A cardiovascular problem, high blood pressure, and/or lipid abnormalities are warning signs of an underlying metabolic problem and a glucose/insulin abnormality called **cardio metabolic risk**.

can you catch diabetes?

You don't catch diabetes. It's not something going around. The roots of diabetes are in your DNA, which is why your chances for avoiding it are easily compromised by poor lifestyle decisions. Your genes determine how the cells that make up your organs and body systems will operate. This genetic blueprint is often referred to as the human genotype.

Diabetes is actually a genetic disorder, which means your genes carry a variation or mutation. Usually, these mutated genes make you vulnerable to all sorts of diseases. For example, having mutations to certain genes can predispose you to developing cancer if you also smoke or are exposed to toxins in the workplace.

Some genetic disorders are inherited. A mutated gene passed down through a family means each generation can inherit the gene that causes a disease. Still other genetic disorders are due to problems in chromosomes comprising a chain of genes. For example, in certain birth defects, such as Down's syndrome, the child has an extra copy of one chromosome. A family history of diabetes is a risk factor for the disease. You need to tell your children that if other family members, especially parents and grandparents, have diabetes, they are likely to develop diabetes, too. You all must be aware of this most important threat to future health. It's critical to keep in mind that if you develop diabetes, or are at risk because it's part of your genetic code, how you live is extra important.

You can beat the genetic odds by proper lifestyle, weight loss, and compliance with medication plans. If you have a family medical history of diabetes, you can have more empowerment over the disease than others who have just discovered they have prediabetes. Your physician or nurse will ask for your medical history, including childhood and adolescent medical problems and any acute health problems—even the flu. Your physician should counsel you on your diabetes risk. If he or she doesn't do so, you should request it. And you should begin to educate yourself on this disease immediately.

One of the oddest aspects of diabetes is that many medical professionals as well as laypeople think it is easy to diagnose with a blood test. This is another roadblock because the doctor may only look for diabetes, not concomitant diseases that many people with prediabetes and diabetes have. You may have had diabetes for several years because diabetes can often be asymptomatic, which is *not* the same as dormant. Unless you recognize that you have unexplained symptoms and are not feeling well, by the time a specialist orders a full panel of tests, your diabetes may have progressed significantly.

Even the methods of diagnosis described later in this chapter can affect weight loss because each patient is different, but not all are treated individually. Your physician may prescribe the same medications for patients who have different baseline test results. If you are underdiagnosed and you have been told that you only have prediabetes, your chances of weight loss are vastly diminished. Many people actually do receive a stronger message from their doctors, but they put a more positive spin on their diagnosis to avoid dealing with the truth.

Type 2 diabetes is a complex disorder that starts with your genetic makeup. It affects your endocrine system as you grow, and diabetes ultimately leads to cardiovascular disaster if you don't halt its progression. This is why understanding your diabetes is the key to your weight loss and why early diagnosis and individualized treatment are so critical.

your diabetic potential: the big three

The following three factors increase the likelihood that you will develop prediabetes or type 2 diabetes.

1. Visceral adiposity (belly fat): a waistline larger than 40 inches (1 m) in men and 35 inches (88.9 cm) in women.
2. A high level of triglycerides
3. A family history of diabetes

If you have all three factors, you are ten times more likely to develop diabetes than someone without all of these conditions. You may also have a **hypertriglyceridemic waist**, which is the presence of belly fat and high triglycerides, that suggests you're at risk for *both* heart disease and diabetes.

Even though lack of health education, denial, and self-deception may have led to the epidemic of diabetes we face, this epidemic has prompted considerable successful research and a better understanding of the link between diabetes, cardiovascular disease, and a cluster of symptoms that contribute to weight gain and poor health (i.e., metabolic syndrome). With this understanding, patients have been able to more successfully manage their disease themselves. This is important for weight loss because while the stats alone don't sound promising, diabetes and weight loss are strongly influenced by the patient's efforts.

WATCH FOR SYMPTOMS

Especially if you have a family history of diabetes, you must watch out for the following diabetes warning signs:

- Frequent urination
- Increased thirst (and water does not usually help)
- Changes in appetite
- Diminished energy level and fatigue
- Blurred vision
- Unexplained weight loss
- Numbness and tingling in your hands and feet
- Cuts or wounds that take longer to heal
- Falling asleep after eating
- Erectile dysfunction in men
- Frequent urinary tract infections

People with type 2 diabetes might have a condition called silent ischemia, which is having a significant coronary obstruction (severe lack of blood flow) without chest pain. You can even have a heart attack without having chest pain. This condition can also occur in nondiabetics.

Ignoring these symptoms or ascribing them to another cause is the worst thing you can do. If you have diabetes, a battle is raging in your body that may have already been provoked by risk factors, such as your family history, age, sex, ethnic background, undiagnosed hypertension, high cholesterol and other uncontrolled lipid levels, and even giving birth to a baby weighing more than 9 pounds (4.1 kg).

UNDERSTAND THE SUGAR CONNECTION

Diabetes is not a simple disease caused by what people think is the "sugar" or glucose level in their bloodstreams. Diabetes is usually much more complicated, creating havoc with your organs and vascular system. Compare your disease to a line of twisters moving through a town, flattening buildings left and right, except that your disease has been silently doing its damage over the course of many years.

People with diabetes often say, "My sugar is high (or low)," as if they've put too much sugar in their coffee or on their cereal. This myth is another common roadblock to weight loss. As a diabetic, your problem is not the same as too much of that granular stuff in the little bags. The sugar to which diabetics refer is **glucose**, the fuel-like product generated in the body as it breaks food into its essential components: fats, carbohydrates, protein, minerals, and vitamins. Glucose is absorbed into the bloodstream, where it is transported to receptor sites in your organs and muscles to be used for energy.

Insulin plays a key role in this process. Your body manufactures it naturally, but when the body doesn't make enough insulin or stops making it altogether, synthetic insulin is used to treat type 2 diabetes in the later stages. When you eat, much of your food is converted to glucose. Insulin is manufactured by the **beta cells** of your pancreas and transported through the bloodstream to your cells, which allows the glucose to be metabolized into energy for daily activities.

You will often hear about something called **insulin resistance**, which is a very important concept in diabetes. Simply put, insulin resistance is when the normal level of insulin produced by your pancreas does not enable glucose to enter the cells normally, as per their genetic programming. The result is a message sent back to the pancreas, which responds by generating more insulin. When the body cells still do not respond to the insulin and continue to resist, glucose (too much sugar) builds up in the blood.

To put it another way, insulin resistance is a diminished ability of organs to take up and metabolize glucose in response to the higher level of insulin. You can think of it as a relative lack of insulin that actually works. This situation is especially common where visceral adiposity exists. Although your bloodstream and the insulin receptor sites in your body are already overflowing with insulin, the body's cells carry out their normal signaling duty, telling the pancreas that your insulin is not working. As a result, your pancreas produces more insulin, raising the overall level in the bloodstream and leading to a condition called **hyperinsulinemia** because the high insulin levels that result are now toxic to the body.

Insulin resistance, prediabetes, and type 2 diabetes are linked because your muscles, fat, and liver are not using insulin as intended. As noted, the pancreas keeps striving to meet the call for more insulin by sending more out. In the long run, excess glucose builds up in the bloodstream, circulating and keeping you in a state of insulin resistance.

A real danger to your health can result from all of this. The repeated demand on the pancreas to produce insulin in the face of excessive calories, high blood sugar, and excessive carbohydrate intake with insulin resistance puts a mounting burden on the beta cells, which is a condition that I call **beta cells stress syndrome**.

Pancreatic beta cell burnout finally occurs when the pancreas decreases the amount of insulin it produces, and the diabetic now requires insulin replacement therapy. This is why most people with type 2 diabetes, especially longstanding diabetes, require insulin. The beta cell failure is intensified by high glucose and fat levels in the blood, called lipotoxicity and glycotoxicity.

People with blood glucose levels that are higher than normal but not yet in the diabetic range have prediabetes. Doctors sometimes call this condition impaired fasting glucose (IFG) or impaired glucose tolerance (IGT), depending on the test used to diagnose it. Prediabetes is becoming more common in the United States, according to new estimates provided by the U.S. Department of Health and Human Services. In 2000, about 40 percent of U.S. adults ages 40 to 74—or 41 million people—had prediabetes. New data suggest that at least 57 million U.S. adults had prediabetes in 2002.

early diagnosis is critical

Research into the pathophysiology (the study of disturbances of normal body functions) of type 2 diabetes indicates that "by the time a diabetic is diagnosed, the patient has lost 80 percent of beta cell function, and an individual with impaired fasting glucose (prediabetic) has lost up to 50 percent of his beta cell volume," according to the American Diabetes Association.

Unfortunately, until recently prediabetes was not considered dangerous by many patients, and doctors didn't treat it aggressively. This situation is beginning to change.

If you have prediabetes, you have a higher risk of developing type 2 diabetes, formerly called adult-onset diabetes or non-insulin-dependent diabetes. According to studies by the National Diabetes Information Clearing House, National Institutes of Health, most people with prediabetes go on to develop type 2 diabetes within 10 years, unless they lose 5 to 7 percent of their body weight—which is about 10 to 15 pounds (4.5 to 6.8 kg) for someone who weighs 200 pounds (90.7 kg)—by making modest changes in their diet and level of physical activity. People with prediabetes also have a higher risk of heart disease.

As you will learn in Step Three: Nutrition, the types of foods you eat affect the amount of glucose that goes into your bloodstream and the speed with which it does so. In case of carbohydrates, many affect our blood glucose level differently. These foods are listed on something called the glycemic index (GI), which can help you choose foods that reduce insulin resistance. The GI expresses them in a range—those with lower numbers being healthier. An example would be certain vegetables, whole grains, legumes, and nuts. The glycemic index can be found in many books, and on websites including www.glycemicindex.com.

Highly processed foods, such as sugared cereals, require very little digestive activity. Your body converts them to glucose with minimal effort. Complex carbohydrates, such as those found in whole grain pasta or whole grains, digest more slowly and result in a less rapid rise in blood sugar. The longer you have to burn the carbohydrates, the better off you are. The glucose from them will enter your system over a longer period of time, so your body will be able to metabolize it properly.

UNDERSTAND THE LINK BETWEEN DIABETES AND OBESITY

For the past few decades, it has become obvious that there is a very real epidemic in the United States of obesity linked directly to insulin dysfunction, or diabetes, that poses grave risk for the heart. Scientists call this condition **diabesity**. The term came about because of the link between the two.

Diabetes has often been thought of as only an endocrine disorder. However, because of the high incidence of cardiovascular diseases that follow in its wake, it is now classified differently by many doctors. The new definition of diabetes also characterizes it as a cardiovascular disease—a significant roadblock.

The endocrine system, composed of glands, helps control virtually all bodily functions as it dispenses hormones that journey to the bloodstream to dock with the specific body system that requires the hormone. Hormones affect your moods, your ability to reproduce, and the work of organs such as the pancreas.

The weight gain connection to the activities of the endocrine system is clear: If your blood sugar drops and you eat a sweet or starch, your blood sugar will rise sharply and then drop again after the insulin converts it to fuel. The fluctuations in glucose and insulin levels lead to hunger, craving, and bingeing. You have no metabolic stability.

From a biological perspective, how much weight you gain in the process is secondary to this hormonal dysregulation and the associated problems of diabetes. In reality, it's all a vicious circle—you're tired; your legs or your joints hurt so you can't exercise, or you can't exercise because you have low testosterone; or you can't get out of the chair because your sugar is 200 to 300; after you eat a heavy meal, you're tired … and on it goes.

The new view of diabetes as both an endocrine disorder and a cardiovascular disease significantly changes how you should be diagnosed and treated, especially if you must lose weight. Many studies now indicate that more people with type 2 diabetes die from myocardial infarctions—heart attack—than the general population. Additionally, all forms of cardiovascular disease, strokes, and their complications cause many deaths among people with diabetes. More than 50 percent of people with diabetes will eventually succumb to heart disease.

The risk of coronary heart disease in women with diabetes is significantly higher than it is in men with diabetes. In the Nurses Health Study, conducted in the 1970s and 1980s and involving more than 100,000 women, scientists found that women who eventually developed diabetes also were at a significantly elevated risk of heart attack and stroke prior to the diagnosis of diabetes. The signs of risk of cardiovascular disease began at least fifteen years before the diagnosis of diabetes.

According to the American Diabetes Association (ADA), "Several studies have indicated that classic cardiovascular complications are frequently present at the

prediabetes: the ticking clock

In preventive medicine, scientists and practitioners search for the causes of disease. In a study of Korean War soldiers fifty-five years ago, scientists were surprised to find the beginnings of cardiovascular disease in these young men, as well as significant coronary artery disease. Today, scientists have identified cardiovascular risk factors in children, and a number of recent studies report that the onset of diabetes can be detected long before a confirmed diagnosis of diabetes is reached.

This phenomenon is called "the ticking clock." The *San Antonio Heart Study*, conducted in the 1980s and 1990s, found that many people with identifiable heart disease risk factors turned out to develop diabetes in the course of the fifteen-year study. Recent medical research has reaffirmed the strong connection between elevated glucose levels (hyperglycemia) and heart disease. In addition to recent studies by the American Diabetes Association, the prestigious British medical journal *The Lancet* published a study in August 2008 found that people who suffer a heart attack are three to four more times as likely to be diagnosed with prediabetes or diabetes. The conclusions in the study were based on new guidelines for diagnosing prediabetes and diabetes. The latter have not yet been universally used by the medical community, and as a result there is some confusion about the diagnosis of diabetes, especially when it comes to blood glucose levels.

diagnosis of type 2 diabetes." Many times, cardiac complications or problems are discovered and then the patients are also found to have prediabetes or type 2 diabetes. This was not recognized prior to cardiovascular symptoms or diagnosis. The ADA adds that the conventional risk factors for heart disease "contribute similarly to the macrovascular (large vessel) and microvascular (small vessel) complications in type 2 diabetes." In addition, these risk factors, present at the diagnosis of heart disease along with asymptomatic atherosclerosis (i.e., buildup of plaque in the arteries), are "associated with insulin resistance."

Diabetic heart disease, which is another condition often found in people with diabetes, is due to fatty infiltration of the myocardium or heart. Increasingly, obesity as a diabetic and as a heart patient is linked to blood vessels carrying triglyceride-rich blood and fat that infiltrates the heart and liver. These fatty deposits in the liver are common in obese people, diabetics, and prediabetics. New research shows that the fat is also deposited in the pancreas.

This connection between insulin and heart disease is also a key aspect of **metabolic syndrome**, which is the cluster of biological symptoms described earlier that includes glucose abnormalities, hypertension, high triglycerides, and "central obesity" (the pear shape or prominent belly that many people have). A report from the proceedings of the European Heart Society Congress offers evidence of this connection in a study that found women with hypertension to be three times as likely to develop diabetes than were women without hypertension. Further, data suggest that many individuals with any type of heart ailment, be it a heart attack, stroke, peripheral vascular disease, angioplasty or bypass surgery experience, hypertension, or hyperlipidemia, will be found upon closer examination to have elevated glucose levels indicative of undiagnosed prediabetes or diabetes.

WATCH OUT FOR AN EXPANDING WAISTLINE

Many people look through family albums to find their pictures from high school or college. Did you look thin and fit? Could you still fit into that outfit you were wearing? Do you now hide in the back row when someone takes family pictures? This behavior is one of those nonscientific signs that you may be becoming insulin resistant, and you may have put yourself on track for one of the more overlooked indicators of diabetes that is as significant as any blood test.

While insulin resistance is definitely a part of prediabetes and type 2 diabetes, visceral adiposity (VA) is not really just the roll of fat that circles your waist, or even subcutaneous fats. Visceral fat is considered to be an endocrine organ

visceral adipose causes and complications

What causes visceral adiposity (VA)? Genetics, compounded by poor lifestyle choices.

What are its complications? There is also a significant link between VA and cardiovascular disease, which confirms the link between heart disease and weight gain. Left untreated, hyperglycemia-damaged nerves and blood vessels, enhanced by VA, can lead to heart disease, stroke, kidney disease, blindness, diabetic neuropathy, gum infections, and gangrene.

itself, and it cannot be mentioned too many times is a primary link to diabetes and as an agent of weight gain.

VA is composed of a specific type of body fat—adipose tissue—that normally functions as a fuel storage tank. Adipose tissue is found at various sites throughout the body, including the waist, to keep you warm, to cushion bones from falls, and to store energy reserves. When you exercise, you lose weight because you use stored fuel drawn from adipose fat. Excessive adipose tissue is why overweight people often complain that they feel hot.

The presence of VA is usually determined by an equation involving the circumference of your waistline, the circumference of your hips, the volume of intra-abdominal fat, and other factors. Few people with diabetes do not have VA. Visceral adiposity exists in children and adolescents, and a child who has both high triglycerides and a family history of diabetes is as much at risk as his parents are for both diabetes and heart disease. Reports in the media, such as a recent article in the *Wall Street Journal*, cite scientific studies that a higher than ever percentage of adolescents are now taking cholesterol and blood pressure drugs and are developing diabetes. This suggests that children are increasingly developing what previously had been an adult disorder: metabolic syndrome.

KNOW ABOUT THE DAMAGE DONE BY UNTREATED HIGH BLOOD GLUCOSE LEVELS

To understand just how important preventing diabetic progression is, you should be aware of the conditions that are caused by untreated, chronically elevated glucose and acute after-meal high blood glucose, which is called **postprandial hyperglycemia**. These prediabetic conditions damage nerve tissue and blood vessels, and they also increase the risk of cardiovascular disease, accelerating the aging process.

This doesn't mean that you'll find more wrinkles sooner or that you'll begin to walk stooped over. The aging process is more insidious. Here are the conditions caused by untreated high blood glucose level:

- Hyperglycemia causes twice the risk of a heart attack and lipids will rise, leading to more premature coronary vessel disease. In fact, with diabetes, most diseases usually associated with aging, such as hypertension, blood vessel disease, and kidney disease, also appear.

- Severe damage caused by hyperglycemia has been implicated in endothelial dysfunction (abnormalities in the inner lining of the blood vessels, which is very important to cardiovascular health); this can lead to hypertension and accelerated arteriosclerosis.
- Hyperglycemia can also worsen oxidative stress, which is damage to the tissues, organs, and blood vessels from oxidation.
- Inflammatory changes in the body caused by hyperglycemia have been associated with accelerated heart disease and aging. The body's response to cell damage is a known risk factor in cardiovascular disease. It is marked by high levels of C-reactive protein (CRP) or cardio-CRP, which raises heart disease risk, and fibrinogen (a clotting factor), and white blood cell count in the blood.
- High glucose levels can also be responsible for glycosylation, the process in which glucose bonds with proteins and lipids. Glycosylation is extremely dangerous because it accelerates the production of advanced glycation end-products (AGEs). AGEs are by-products of high sugar that attach to proteins and DNA, leading to increased blood vessel, nerve, and tissue damage.
- A high glucose level leads to poor lipid control. Years ago, cholesterol became a household word through the educational efforts of the National Cholesterol Education Program of the Institutes of Medicine. Today, poor lipid control is known to be as important a risk factor for heart disease as cholesterol (hyperlipidemia) is, yet it is not given sufficient attention by medical practitioners. High glucose levels result is what is sometimes called the atherogenci and thrombogenic lipid profiles. This profile consists of high triglycerides, low HDL, increased small particle size LDL, and changes in blood clotting characteristics.
- Untreated high glucose can also cause **thrombosis**. Coronary thrombosis, or the forming of blood clots in the heart, can cause heart attacks.
- Associated problems are **postprandial hyperglycemia** (elevated glucose after meals) and **postprandial hyperlipidemia** (elevated lipids after meals). These problems are referred to as **postprandial dysmetabolism** (defective metabolism)—elevated glucose and fats after meals that may contribute to an acute heart attack and sudden death.
- Continued elevated blood sugar is one of the reasons cuts or infections heal slower for a diabetic.

- People with diabetes with poor glucose control are prone to various levels of nerve damage, or **neuropathy**. This shows up as numbness, tingling and loss of feeling, particularly in the extremities, and it can be disabling.

- Elevated blood glucose also can lead to **peripheral vascular disease** (PVD), which diminishes the ability of blood vessels in the head, hands, feet, arms, and legs to carry oxygen to the cells and remove waste products in these tissues, resulting in serious foot and vision problems. After traumatic accidents, diabetes is the second most common cause of foot and leg amputations in men and women.

- Men are more likely than women to develop PVD because of higher levels of smoking and treatment resistance, but women who smoke substantially increase the likelihood that they will develop PVD. In addition to impaired circulation, PVD causes muscle aches and cramps, characterized by pain in the legs when walking that eases with rest. It can occur in the calves, thighs, and buttocks, depending on the location of arterial blockages.

- For people with diabetes of either sex, kidney disease can develop slowly over a number of years, leading to a devastating result. More than a one-third of all new victims of end-stage renal disease are diabetic. In end-stage renal disease, or **diabetic nephropathy**, the main early symptom is increased urinary protein (albumin). Often, people with diabetes with kidney disease spend several hours, multiple times per week on dialysis machines to cleanse their blood. Some require kidney transplants.

You can see how important it is to deal with your glucose and insulin levels quickly and to be aware of ancillary problems beyond the ones listed above, including hypertension, and hormone (especially thyroid and sex hormone) dysfunction. If these conditions occur, the roadblocks to health grow even higher.

Additional conditions that can complicate treatment and that must be addressed include visceral adiposity; elevated levels of homocystine (an amino acid that increases risk of vascular disease) in the blood elevated levels of uric acid in the urine, and progressive nerve and vascular problems, including retinal and renal disorders. These problems have to come under an all-out attack at some point in your treatment that may include drug and natural therapies plus a totally dedicated lifestyle change.

take control

Studies have shown that even in people with overall good glucose management but intermittent elevation of glucose, acute hypergycemia causes damaging effects. For that reason, it's even more important that you control prediabetes. For example, it is now suggested that the fasting blood sugar levels have to be even lower than 90.

Controlling high blood sugar helps prevent heart disease, strokes, kidney disease, circulation problems, and blindness. Diabetes is the leading cause of amputations, blindness, and renal failure leading to dialysis in the United States.

Understanding all of this information should not frighten you. It can make staying on a weight loss course less difficult. This does not mean the process will be simple, nor will medication magically heal you. The task isn't easy because as a prediabetic or diabetic, you are holding back the flood while trying to change your life.

HAVE A DIABETIC WORKUP: THE LAST AND MOST IMPORTANT STEP IN EDUCATION

The Five-Step Plan is a comprehensive program, and you will only succeed if you embrace all aspects of it. Proper diagnosis is a critical part of this weight loss plan—in-depth knowledge of your own condition. This section outlines and explains the kind of examination you should undergo to determine your health status before starting in on Step One and the rest of the five steps.

In short, it is a complete medical exam and metabolic workup. Who should be giving it to you?

Choosing a Doctor

If you have a diabetic problem, the right physician is going to become your new BFF—best friend forever, as the kids say. No matter how frequently you go to the doctor's office, you will have to respect each other and partner-up in your care. Ultimately, you will need to have total faith in him or her and be willing to put your life in his or her hands, especially in a comprehensive, roadblock-destroying weight loss plan.

If you have diabetes, this is likely to be a specialist. In my case, my family physician, whom I had seen for many years, decided that my high glucose levels, elevated cholesterol, and blood pressure all indicated that I should see a cardiologist and diabetologist. In retrospect, she was very smart: She also diagnosed my denial and lack of motivation to change my health behavior. By sending me to a specialist, she recognized that, in the hands of someone who dealt with patients like me daily, there was a chance for me. She was right, and she likely saved my life.

Most people end up in a specialist's office when someone, perhaps your primary physician, gives them a referral name. Is it that simple or even a good idea to make your choice this way? You may have to because of your insurance rules. Also, your choice depends on whether a recommended doctor accepts your insurance. The reality is there are many doctors who work in group practices who spread their patients around because they simply don't have time to see any more patients. Further, some HMO rules actually set the number of patients a physician has to see every day. In addition, doctors cannot accept your insurance if they are not in your network; it's illegal.

Sometimes if you can't get the doctor you've been referred to, it can be a blessing in disguise. First, doctors within a practice consult with each other all of the time. In hospital-based practices, which are very common, you may end up with a younger doctor who actually has more time to spend with individual patients, and that is in your favor when it comes to both treatment and accessibility.

While professional referral is the most common way of finding a doctor, many specialists get a large percentage of their patients from word-of-mouth recommendations. Even though this is the way many people find a doctor, it is not always the best way. However, it can be a good choice if the person who gave you the name is an "original source," an actual patient.

Here's a few more ways to find a doctor:

- Lists of specialists are available from the American Board of Medical Specialists (800-776-2378) and other organizations, such as the American Diabetes Association (www.diabetes.org) and the American Heart Association (www.americanheart.org).

- Ancillary health-care professionals can be a good source of referrals. Many diabetes and cardiac patients spend considerable time with physical therapists, nutritionists, and other members of rehab/diet programs. They can be excellent sources of information and suggestions.
- A local hospital can provide names of staff cardiologists and connect you to people in its cardiovascular program.
- Many medical practices and virtually every hospital or clinic has a website. Spend some time online looking at both the doctor's credentials and information about the facility.

In the end, how do you make this choice that is so important to your treatment? Keep the following in mind:
- You want to find a doctor who has as much hands-on experience as possible.
- If you have diabetes, you want a doctor who has, or has access to, a good diet, nutrition, and exercise approach to care.
- Many doctors do not have a good health education system tailored for people with prediabetes or diabetes. Find someone who does and who you can access for information you need.

When choosing a doctor, it might be helpful to ask the following questions:
- Is the doctor conservative or aggressive in his approach?
- Is the practice affiliated with a hospital you'd want to go to if necessary?
- Do you like the doctor? If you don't, your motivation to comply with a treatment plan might be undone.
- Does this doctor inspire you to regain your health?
- Do you feel comfortable going to the doctor's office?
- Does the doctor's style fit your personality?
- Does the doctor listen to you and does he or she respond to you? Don't hesitate to let a doctor know when you don't understand something.
- Does the doctor respectfully answer all of your questions, regardless of their origin, such as the Internet or a family member?

Always make sure to ask for your medical records from your primary care doctor before your appointment and bring them and the results of your blood tests to the diabetes specialist.

- Can you get to the office easily for regular visits?
- Do you have to spend hours waiting in the office on a regular basis? (This could indicate that the doctor is overbooked or the staff is not responding to you. However, the practice of medicine today is filled with paperwork and forms that can stretch a staff's capabilities.)
- Does the staff willingly help you correctly fill out the paperwork?
- What are the doctor's views on alternative therapies and how do they compare with yours?
- Does the doctor have a wide circle of relationships with others who can help you if a certain procedure is required?

It's important to choose your doctor wisely, but keep in mind that there is no reason that you cannot change doctors if and when necessary. After all, your health is at stake.

Getting a Complete Medical Exam

Many of us no longer go for an annual physical unless it's required for work or insurance. However, to lose weight as a prediabetic or diabetic, you must have a complete total-body physical exam, along with the blood tests listed on page 52. I consider this the initial aspect of the steps that will be discussed in the following chapters, because without an in-depth look at you from the inside out, your decisions will not be informed ones.

The following describes all that the exam should include. If yours is not as thorough as this, ask your physician why it is not.

think ahead

Before your appointment, call the doctor's office and ask for a copy of the family and medical history forms and fill them out. The forms are important, and you may have to call some relatives to get full and correct information. A crowded, noisy waiting room is not the place to do this.

Many medical practices have these forms on their websites, or the office staff can send them to you via email or regular mail. Check my website (www.drvagnini.com) for more information.

Your Medical History

The first thing that you should be asked to do is complete a standard medical history form. This gives the physician a basic picture of your past health conditions, but remember, it's called "standard" for a reason: It does not necessarily cover your full medical history.

To create a diabetic weight loss program that meets your unique needs, you and your physician need a complete picture of your current and past family medical history. A partial list of information that you will be asked to provide follows. The complete recommended form is on the Five-Step Plan website www.drvagnini.com. If your doctor doesn't ask for this amount of information, complete the form here and take a copy of it to your appointment. Your doctor will thank you!

General cardiovascular/diabetes history:

- Arteriosclerosis
- Stroke
- Aneurysm
- Heart attack
- Peripheral arterial disease
- Prediabetes
- Type 2 diabetes
- Type 1 diabetes

Cardiac-specific history:

- Chest pain
- Angina
- History of heart attack
- Hypertension
- Coronary bypass surgery
- Coronary angioplasty
- Shortness of breath
- Arrhythmia
- Palpitations
- Rheumatic fever
- Pain in the throat on exertion
- Ankle edema

- Sleeping on more than two pillows (The inability to lie flat in bed without becoming breathless can indicate heart or lung problems.)
- Cardiovascular problems
- Congenital heart disease
- Mitral valve prolapse
- Being awakened by shortness of breath
- Sleep apnea

General cerebrovascular and cardiac peripheral vascular conditions:
- Smoking
- Overweight
- High blood pressure
- Diabetes
- High cholesterol
- High triglycerides
- High LDL
- Previous heart attack
- Irregular heartbeat
- Shortness of breath

Any hospitalizations and surgeries:

Your current medications and dosages:

Family medical history: (For each, this should include hypertension, diabetes, arteriosclerosis, heart attack, stroke, kidney disease, tuberculosis, and thyroid disease.)
- Mother
- Father
- Grandparents
- Siblings
- Aunts and uncles

Your social history:
- Marital status
- Birthplace

- Foreign travels
- Daily caffeine consumption
- Daily alcohol consumption
- Stress
- Activity level

Overall review of your health:
- Results of electrocardiogram
- Weakness
- Fatigue
- Chills
- Fever
- Night sweats
- Sleeping problems
- Phobias
- Appetite
- Food intolerances
- Respiratory, skin, or environmental allergies

Central nervous system conditions:
- Headache
- Dizzy spells
- Lightheadedness
- Convulsions
- Blacking out

Respiratory conditions:
- Cough
- Pneumonia
- Chronic bronchitis
- Chronic obstructive pulmonary disease and asthma

Peripheral vascular conditions:
- Pain in legs after walking (calves/thighs/buttocks)
  - Leg or arm pain
  - Leg cramps

- Tightness in legs
- Varicose veins
- Cold hands or feet
- Numbness in hands or feet
- Heaviness in legs

Other general health issues:

- Transient ischemic attacks (TIAs) or mini-strokes
- Ear problems
- Eye problems
- Nose, throat, and sinus problems
- Nosebleeds
- Teeth problems
- Breast problems
- Gastrointestinal problems
- Urinary tract pain or infection
- Musculoskeletal problems
- Endocrine problems

Psychiatric issues:

- Anxiety attacks
- Depression
- Other mental problems

This may seem like a lot of information for you to provide, but all of your answers help your doctor in the following two ways:

1. Your doctor will have a complete picture of your overall history of medical problems.
2. With this information, your doctor can better focus on symptoms you may indicate. For example, breathlessness in a diabetic can indicate silent angina and the presence of heart disease.

know your numbers

Health knowledge is essential as the basis for personal health maintenance—with an eye toward longevity. You may not get all these numbers right in a pop quiz, but it is important to know of them and that they are key indicators of the state of your health. Here's some basic information.

Blood pressure: The first thing your health-care provider does when you visit is take your blood pressure, because blood pressure levels tell much about your health condition at any moment in time. A healthy blood pressure had been considered in the range of 120 to 140 mmhg (millimeters of mercury) in the systolic (top number) and below 90 mmhg in the diastolic (bottom number). New guidelines are blood pressure below 135/85 and lower than 120/80 for people with renal impairment. Abnormally high blood pressure is a clue that something unhealthy is going on in the body. When blood pressure is chronically high, it is a condition called **hypertension**, which requires aggressive treatment, because it can lead to very serious health problems, such as stroke or heart attack. Ask your doctor how you can monitor your blood pressure at home.

Total cholesterol: The National Cholesterol Education Program, a program of the National Health Institutes, publishes recommended cholesterol levels for maintaining low risk of health problems, specifically cardiovascular health. A measurement below 200 mg/dl (milligrams per deciliter of blood) is the desirable level that puts you at lower risk for coronary heart disease. If your total cholesterol number is not below 200, ask your doctor how to get it down there!

High-density lipoprotein (HDL) cholesterol: This is known as the "good" cholesterol, which you can remember by thinking of "H" as healthy. This specific type of cholesterol acts to remove unhealthy deposits in the artery wall and is therefore felt to be very cardio protective. Women have the good fortune of genetically high HDL. Levels higher than 40 mg/dl are considered good. You can increase your HDL with exercise, taking niacin, and lowering tryglycerides.

Low-density cholesterol (LDL) is reported as the "bad" cholesterol. This type of lipid, when oxidized, adheres to the blood vessel wall, setting up an inflammatory cascade leading to arteriosclerotic plaque deposition. Recent research has advised maintaining an LDL at 100 mg/dl or below. Newer research suggests that people with heart or blood vessel disease should reduced their LDL to below 70. This intensive lipid lowering has been shown to reverse arteriosclerotic disease.

Triglycerides are another type of fat in the blood. This is just as important as cholesterol. A good level for triglycerides is 150 mg or below. Testing should be done after an eight- to twelve-hour fast. Elevations usually occur in people with metabolic syndrome, abdominal obesity, prediabetes, and diabetes. Elevation is also associated with high sugar and high dietary intake.

Fasting plasma glucose (FPG): This is the measure of glucose (sugar) in the blood, which is a test for diabetes. It is measured in blood drawn after an eight-hour (usually overnight) fast. Diabetes is indicated when the glucose level in the blood is over 126 mg/dl. That is, the body's metabolism is not able to process glucose in the blood sufficiently. Levels of 100 to 125 are considered to be impaired glucose tolerance (IGT) or prediabetes. Diabetes is indicated if the glucose level of the blood is over 125. Recent research has revealed that fasting levels of 90 to 100 probably represent prediabetes as well.

Homocysteine: In medical science's ongoing effort to discover what causes people to have heart attacks, it has identified a number biochemical factors; one of them is homocysteine. This is a kind of amino acid produced naturally, but it has been found at high levels in persons who have heart disease. Current standards regard a homocysteine level below 16 mg/dl in the blood as desirable. When levels are higher than 16, efforts should be made to reduce it, mainly by taking dietary supplements, such as folic acid and vitamins B_6 and B_{12}, riboflavin, garlic, and omega-3 fatty acids. Elevation of homocystine is very common in people with diabetes.

High-sensitivity C-reactive protein (CRP): This is a protein in the blood that is present when inflammation occurs in the body, including inflammation in the coronary arteries that is associated with heart disease. A measure below 3 mg/L (milligrams per liter) is considered a safe level. A level of 3 and greater indicates risk and calls for additional testing and treatment.

Complete Blood/Metabolic Analysis

The initial profile that your physician draws from your medical history form is really the proverbial tip of the iceberg. For a more complete picture of your total health, a series of blood and other tests will be perfomed to develop a complete metabolic profile. These tests will be added to the growing portrait of your health and combined will begin to indicate what your optimum diet approach may be.

This series of tests might require that you have the same tests at different times. Some can be done in a walk-in lab in your community, and others require that you be monitored for a specific period of time in the doctor's office. Some of these tests may require fasting and will likely be done in the early morning. You will be given tests that measure potential for diabetes, heart disease, and anything else your doctor suspects may be present, based on your family and personal medical history.

Recommended blood chemistry tests: Extensive blood chemistries are important for diagnosing and managing prediabetes, diabetes, and cardiovascular problems. I recommend you have the following tests:

- Diabetic testing, including fasting glucose, insulin level, hemoglobin A1C, and C peptide (see pages 53–55.)
- Comprehensive metabolic profiles, including protein and albumin levels in the blood, kidney function, liver function, electrolytes, uric acid, and serum iron
- A complete blood count, including differentials in white blood cell counts
- Urinalysis with microalbumin
- Comprehensive thyroid profile with thyroid-stimulating hormone test (TSH), thyroid antibodies when indicated or when there is suspicion of autoimmune thyroid disease
- Arthritis panel for autoimmune, rheumatoid factor, and Lyme disease in people with arthritis
- Comprehensive lipid profile, including cholesterol, HDL, LDL, and triglycerides
- Lipid fractionation, including LDL particle size and total LDL count (This is extremely important for risk stratification.)
- Lipoprotein-associated phospholipase A2 (Lp-PLA2), which measures the specific enzyme in the blood that occurs during an active atherosclerotic process that could lead to rupture of plaque and cause sudden heart attack or stroke

- Homocysteine level
- Coagulation profile with fibrinogen
- Vitamin B_{12}, folic acid, Vitamin D (especially vitamin D_1 and D_2 and the D_2 25-hydroxy, which measures the level of vitamin D_3)
- Gluten sensitivity and food allergy testing, when indicated
- Heavy metals, including mercury, arsenic, lead, and aluminum (This is especially important in view of the recent research indicating high levels of arsenic as related to an increased risk of diabetes. Lead has been shown to increase blood pressure, and mercury is extremely toxic. High mercury levels are quite common in my practice.)
- *Helicobacter pylori* for gastrointestinal problems
- *Candida albicans* for gastrointestinal problems, high-sensitivity C-reactive proteins
- Hormone studies in women, when indicated, including estradiol and progesterone levels
- Hormone studies in men, when indicated, including testosterone levels, PSA (prostate-specific antigen), and DHEA (dehydroepiandrosterone) sulfate
- For people with fatigue, a chronic fatigue profile including titers for Epstein-Barr syndrome, mycoplasma; Lyme disease; herpes 1, 2 and 6; and *Candida albicans*

Blood Testing for Prediabetes and Diabetes

Several blood tests can be used to diagnose diabetes because it is one of the few diseases in which self-management by the patient is critical to his or her survival. Two of the tests are done by a doctor; the other test is done by the patient several times daily.

Blood testing to determine glucose levels is a significant part of diagnosing and managing diabetes when treatment decisions have to be made or modified. However, if you are overweight or obese and must lose weight, these blood tests tell only part of your story. Still, it's important to understand what your doctor is doing and what he is telling you because you will be given, or you will learn to use, one of these blood tests.

Here are the three basic blood tests:

Glucose tolerance test/glucose challenge test: Often called the oral glucose tolerance test, I highly recommend this test and I use it as a diagnostic tool for most of my patients to determine if they are at risk for diabetes, prediabetes, or insulin resistance. This diagnosis, however, includes a family history, presence of obesity, mildly elevated fasting glucose, or metabolic syndrome. The result I found after using this test is that many cases of undiagnosed diabetes are uncovered in my practice.

This test consists of giving an established amount of sugar (6 tablespoons [75 g] in a solution) to a fasting individual. The results have been shown to produce a correct diagnosis in 75 percent of patients whose previous results with other tests have shown only slightly elevated blood sugars. You should discuss this test with your doctor and ask why he or she does not use it. The benefit is that it can give the doctor twice as much of the information he or she needs to accurately diagnose prediabetes or type 2 diabetes and to choose the most appropriate method of treatment.

Generally, the doctor's office sends the test to a laboratory that measures hourly glucose levels and insulin levels. Frequently urine samples are taken, too. By measuring the glucose levels in this manner, your doctor can also often diagnose people who don't have impaired glucose, only elevated insulin levels. These patients can then be treated for their new hyperinsulinemia diagnosis.

You will be asked to fast before this test—usually only water is allowed after midnight the night before the test. At the doctor's office, you will be asked to drink a premeasured liquid that is part glucose.

Your blood will be drawn before drinking the solution and then again at 60-minute intervals after you drink the solution, continuing up to three hours. A diagnosis of diabetes will be based on how high your levels of glucose are above a certain mark. If you are 200 mg/dL at the second hour, you are considered to have diabetes.

A1C test: Today, the most often used diagnostic tool for people with prediabetes and diabetes is a blood test called the hemoglobin A1C. The A1C tests for a blood hemoglobin marker that gives a picture of your average blood glucose for the past three months. Blood is taken every one to three months to determine the level of glucose in the blood over that period. Here's what your A1C numbers mean:

- Normal A1C should be 5.0 mg/dL.
- If the A1C reaches 5.8 mg/dL to 6 mg/dL, it may be indicative of prediabetes, but not under all circumstances.
- An A1C level of 6, representing a three-month average blood glucose of 135 mg/dL, usually indicates type 2 diabetes has developed, but this is not

always the case and should not be used as the sole determinant. Other tests are needed to determine risk factors that might be present.

- Several studies have found that even at A1C levels below 6 mg/dL, there is an increased risk of cardiovascular disease, heart attack, and stroke.
- In the past, the American Diabetic Association indicated that people with diabetes were considered under control at 7 mg/dL or under. New research suggests that the treatment goal should be closer to 6 mg/dL. Recently published research papers have suggested aiming at an even lower level.

One big advantage to using this test is that it does not require that the patient fast before the blood is drawn, and it has been a fairly reliable measurement of blood glucose levels. The test is done in your doctor's office, and it gives you an idea of what your blood sugar levels are over a period of time.

Among its other advantages is that, unlike other blood tests, even if you exercise or diet excessively before the A1C test, it will not change the results.

An objection to using only the A1C test on a patient who is a suspected diabetic is that it can lead to a limited diagnosis. Whenever a patient who presents with symptoms that suggest a diagnosis of diabetes is screened with this blood test, another battery of tests should be done simultaneously to diagnose diabetes, the presence of heart disease, and the level of weight loss required. The misconception that diabetes is a single problem is common. An accurate diagnosis requires more than a simple blood test that is looking only for one answer.

It is extremely important that as a diabetic you get as much information as possible from your physician. Ask your doctor to discuss the metabolic syndrome and your risk of going from prediabetes to diabetes. A diabetes specialist should treat you as someone who also needs cardio-metabolic prevention. Diabetes is a lifelong disease, and your doctor should be treating you not only for today, but also for the future.

Home blood monitoring: You may wonder a why a simple positive or negative test result isn't sufficient for a diagnosis of diabetes. Treatment plans involving a panoply of medications can cause subtle weight gain, which can lead to other problems. You will need to take charge of your disease and monitor how well your new regimen of medications, diet and lifestyle changes, and exercise are working from day to day. Thus, for you as a diagnosed diabetic, daily blood testing with a home blood glucose monitor must become a routine part of your life.

Is your trusty home blood glucose monitoring a possible roadblock to weight loss? Not if you view it as only one aspect of your body's response to the efforts you have been making to overcome diabetes. The device reads the amount of glucose in your blood at a given time and expresses it in terms of milligrams of glucose per deciliter (mg/dL). The meter provides an instant picture—not an average, like the A1C. With the home blood monitor, your blood sugar level readings are specific to different times of day under different circumstances (i.e., fasting, or after meals).

Home blood glucose monitors are sometimes used as a diagnostic test that determines whether you are progressing from prediabetes to full diabetes. Most endocrinologists consider any reading of fasting glucose of 126 or higher as indicative of type 2 diabetes.

The Physical Exam

Earlier, we described the ticking clock concept, which is another reason such an extensive physical workup is required. The tests, when seen as a complete picture, can reveal your hidden risks for diabetes, cardiovascular disease, and metabolic disease. A complete physical examination is an important part of health management for diabetic patients, as well as those with prediabetes or obesity.

In addition to your physical exam, you will be given more tests that measure potential for diabetes, heart disease, and any other medical conditions your doctor suspects may be present, based on your family or personal medical history.

Here's a typical list of these tests:

- Vital signs, including blood pressure in both arms, since a variation in blood pressure above 40 mmHg between the right and left arms could indicate subclavian artery stenosis, which is rare
- Pulse, temperature, and respiratory rate
- Waist measurement
- A 12-lead electrocardiogram and pulmonary function study
- An echocardiogram to determine heart size, heart wall thickness, valve function, and how well your heart muscle can contract
- A cardiac exercise tolerance test, either with echocardiogram or with nuclear imaging to determine cardiac perfusion
- A coronary computer-assisted tomographic (CAT) scan, also called coronary

calcium scoring, which is not be confused with coronary CT angiography, which involves a dye injection that will determine premature or advanced coronary disease (Even in the face of a negative stress test, this should be performed on everyone age fifty and older and on people younger than fifty who are at risk.)

- A retinal exam, preferably with the retina dilated (This is important, and it might be performed by an ophthalmologist. The ophthalmologist also may look at the iris for arcus senilis, a white ring around the iris that may indicate atherosclerosis.)
- Neck examination, including auscultation or placing a stethoscope on the carotid arteries to determine the presence or absence of carotid bruit (an abnormal sound indicating possible arterial narrowing)
- A carotid duplex, which is an ultrasound evaluation of the carotid arteries in the neck (50 percent of strokes are caused by carotid occlusive disease. The lining of the vessels can be measured and followed annually for progression or regression of arteriosclerosis.)
- Abdominal exam, including evaluation for possible abdominal aortic aneurysm, which is difficult to palpate in individuals with excess abdominal fat (An abdominal aortic ultrasound may also be considered to rule out the presence of aneurysm, especially in people with a family history of aneurysm or hypertension.)
- Lower extremity examination
- A sensory examination done with a filament to identify any decreased sensations
- Motor function evaluation by muscle testing and testing of the toes for strength in the lower extremities
- Observation of the skin of the feet and the lower legs, particularly for areas of hair loss indicating a circulatory problem, and dry skin
- Capillary filling (pressing down on the toes to see if they blanch and then fill with blood) and checking for cyanosis (blue or ashy discoloration) and varicose veins, which may indicate a vascular problem
- Examination of the toenails for fungal infections in the toes, which is common in people with diabetes
- Annual evaluation of the peripheral pulses in the blood vessels of the thighs, behind the knees, and two sets of pulses in the feet: one on the top of the foot and one just below the ankle

- A peripheral vascular exam or noninvasive measurement of flows, including an ankle–arm index and ultrasound imaging of the vessels of the lower extremities
- Peripheral nerve test for neuropathy

Receiving Test Feedback: The Moment of Truth

Your doctor should give you an assessment of the findings of the tests described above, starting with any concerns he has about what he found in the routine physical examination, including evidence of circulatory problems, readings of peripheral pulses, and any excess weight.

Then your doctor should thoroughly discuss with you the cardiovascular tests, metabolic markers, and the blood studies, including cholesterol and glucose levels. He or she should explain the results of the glucose tolerance test and indicate whether you have prediabetes, impaired glucose tolerance, impaired fasting glucose, or if you have type 2 diabetes.

The doctor also should explain the importance of hemoglobin A1C and the other risk factors: cholesterol, homocysteine, and C-reactive protein.

This overall evaluation frequently calls for testosterone replacement in men and bioidentical hormone therapy in menopausal women, which uses natural hormone supplements.

By the end of the discussion, you should know exactly how your heart and blood vessels are functioning, what risk factors for diabetes or cardiovascular disease you have, and what you need to bear in mind while organizing and implementing your very own version of the Five-Step Plan.

LOOK AHEAD TO WHAT COMES NEXT

In this chapter, you've learned some of the basics of the clinical definition and management of prediabetes and diabetes and how they affect your potential for weight loss. The most important thing you must remember is that diabetes is not a single disease, and that fact alone might make losing weight a much more difficult task for you. As a result, preventing weight gain and diabetes begins with in-depth health education.

Do you want to prevent diabetes weight gain and its complications and live a longer, healthier life? If so, then this book and its weight loss plan can help save your life. In Step Two, you will learn how medications can change your life and help to control the problems and complications of diabetes and concomitant heart disease. Here's what you will find in the rest of this book:

- You are not getting a diet. You are getting an education and an eating plan that tear down the metabolic roadblocks you face.
- You are going to control your fluctuating glucose and insulin levels that cause food craving and bingeing.
- You are going to control stress and emotional eating.
- You will clear your brain fog by improving overall cardiovascular and metabolic issues, lowering your blood glucose and preventing binge eating.
- You will learn about nutraceuticals, weight loss, and hormone replacement that will end your fatigue.
- You will learn how nutrients work to relieve musculoskeletal problems.
- You will stop postprandial dysmetabolism (defective metabolism after eating), which can be a sign of an association between diabetes and coronary artery disease.
- You will increase your metabolism and thermogenesis, which can help you burn fat and lose weight.
- You will learn to manage or eliminate food allergies.
- You will end your gluten intolerance.
- You will end the gastrointestinal problems associated with obesity, such as dysbiosis (imbalance in the digestive tract), candidiasis, gastroesophageal reflux (GERD), and lack of gastric acid.
- You will overcome your carbohydrate addiction.

In this chapter, you've been exposed to an enormous amount of current research on diabetes and its complications. Now you're ready to take the next step on the path to weight loss and management of your diabetes.

Medications are a critical part of a diabetic weight loss program. Diabetes drugs are not a stand-alone solution for weight loss or glucose control, but they play an extremely important role in achieving your primary goal—diabetes management leading to weight loss.

Medication is listed as Step Two in this plan because losing weight and retaining better overall health are a lot easier when you have prediabetes than when you have full-blown diabetes. Don't forget: Prevention is the key. An important, compelling reason for using medication and taking it properly is that doing so is directly linked to remaining prediabetic or getting back to normal. Further, as a prediabetic or diabetic, your condition is often going to become complicated by several medical conditions that require multiple medications. Through aggressive prediabetic treatment, you can prevent heart attack, stroke, Alzheimer's disease, dementia, certain cancers, and micro or macro vascular disease.

Why is it harder to lose weight when you have diabetes than when you have prediabetes? There's no one thing that makes the process "harder." If you are in an advanced stage of the disease, the metabolic problems are more severe. The roadblocks are more severe.

The more you know about your medications and more faithfully you follow the doctor's orders, the more likely that your diabetes will stay under control. The essence of Step Two, especially for someone with prediabetes, is to prevent progression to diabetes. The right medication is part of an integrated approach to weight loss and diabetes management: restored health, correct medical treatment, and patient/physician cooperation and coordination. As you read on, you will see the result is permanent weight loss.

ARE MEDICATIONS ALWAYS NECESSARY?

Depending on the spectrum of severity with the patients who still have lower levels of glucose, diet, exercise and nutraceuticals are appropriate. With the poorly controlled patients (higher glucose levels) or more obese, more aggressive therapy may be necessary. With the recent paradigm of changes in using multiple medications and considering new research, I generally use drug therapy in both conditions (prediabetes and type 2 diabetes), often prescribing three medications I call "triple therapy": insulin, targeted diet, and exercise.

Can you avoid this? Is it possible to keep your condition under control and avoid weight gain without medication? Yes, but it requires that you focus on prevention at an early stage in your disease. This is one reason why you have learned about the various roadblocks in Step One and the critical importance of prevention. Lifestyle changes can prevent the progression of prediabetes to type 2 diabetes in some patients who are not significantly overweight and who don't have cardiovascular complications. Some of these obstacles can be controlled by diet and lifestyle, but many require medical intervention. Any options you have regarding medication and its effect on weight probably will have been exhausted by the time your doctor brings up the matter of medications.

Consider this: People with prediabetes have only a 50 percent chance of staying that way without medication. By the time you are diagnosed with prediabetes, you have already lost 50 percent of your beta cell function, and your chance of preserving pancreatic function is severely compromised.

Another overall goal of a medication program is to prevent chronic pancreatic/beta cell stress and beta cell burnout. Prevention must begin as soon as possible, so medication may be prescribed for someone with prediabetes. This is why I prefer that most of my patients—even those with prediabetes blood glucose levels—begin drug therapy early even though I am a holistic physician.

Remember, while avoiding the need for medications is possible, it also requires developing a close partnership with your physician and being conscious of what might occur without medication, such as damage to your pancreas, liver, kidneys, heart, and vascular system.

Another important factor to consider is that medications often take time to begin their work. Some medications have a very specific effect, such as aiding weight loss, getting your system back into balance, or slowing down progress of your diabetes.

With a few exceptions, virtually none of the medications described in this chapter are enough to control your diabetes or directly create weight loss in a diabetic. Metformin (brand name Glucophage) and exenatide (brand name Byetta) are those exceptions. Byetta has to be taken at certain times—15 to 60 minutes before eating and is injected through an EpiPen, also known as an auto-injector, for medications that have to be taken quickly or to avoid using syringes.

Another essential component of this program is that you'll need to use nutrients and supplements in addition to your medications, as outlined in the next chapter, and you'll need to be aware of any cardiovascular complications you have. Each step of the overall plan plays an important part in understanding and managing your diabetes. As you learn, your odds of success grow.

PRESCRIBING THE RIGHT MEDICATION FOR YOU

Your diabetologist-physician might have dozens of medical therapies at his or her fingertips, but he or she will rely on clinical experience, current research, and the likelihood of the therapy being effective with your unique medical profile when selecting your medication regimen. Your doctor's judgment of the best treatment for you requires assessment of the severity of your condition when you first see a specialist who treats diabetes. It is critical (and necessary) to the success of your medical treatment that you be under the care of a diabetologist or endocrinologist.

As you read this chapter, keep in mind your doctor's basic goals when choosing your specific diabetes medication. He or she is trying to achieve control of your hyperglycemia (high blood sugar), stop beta cell failure, reduce insulin resistance, reduce visceral fat, reduce inflammation, manage lipid problems and hypertension, reduce antioxidant stress (attacks on the antioxidants that help protect your cells from damage), reduce hypercoagulability (excessive blood clotting), and prevent long-term complications such as eye and nerve damage.

Understanding the benefits and possible side effects of the myriad medications that your doctor might prescribe for you is critical to diabetic weight loss. It is equally important if you have prediabetes or type 2 diabetes or if you are a "combo-diabetic" with complications such as heart or vascular disease. Without clear knowledge of the medications available to you as a diabetic, you will be at a significant disadvantage as you try to reach the goals described above.

It's part of your job as a patient to ask questions and to ensure that your physician is familiar with your entire health picture. Remember that the state of your diabetes is largely in your control once your doctor has you started with a medication. Your doctor prescribes medications to fit your own individual medical profile, so you need to communicate honestly about how the medications are working for you. Keep your doctor in the loop about the side effects of the medication as well.

Communicating with your doctor about your medications is also a crucial step to weight loss in prediabetes. After treatment has begun, you have to keep your bodily functions as close to normal as possible to keep you from gaining more weight. The medications intended to reach this goal (profiled on pages 67–75) can help or hinder you without you knowing it.

As discussed in Step One, multiple blood tests help your physician reduce your risk of disease progression early. However, since diabetes often masks symptoms of heart disease, you must be aggressive about discussing your risks of heart disease with your doctor.

Discuss your entire health picture with your doctor. One medication may help with obesity, but you also may need treatment for high blood pressure and atherosclerosis with other drugs that do not help with weight loss. It's important to understand that medication might be the answer to one metabolic roadblock—

Complicating the pharmaceutical treatment of people with diabetes are their fluctuating glucose and insulin levels, hypertension, lipid abnormalities, and hormone dysfunction, as well as visceral adiposity, homocysteine and uric acid elevation, and progressive nerve and vascular problems, including retinal and renal disorders. These problems must come under an all-out attack that includes drug and natural therapies, plus dedicated lifestyle changes, as described in Step Five.

high glucose levels, for example—but may hamper the effectiveness of medication for treating cardiac problems or hypertension, or vice versa. For example, diuretics and beta-blockers can affect blood glucose levels and may deplete magnesium and vitamin B_1. This is an area to discuss with your doctor; the pros and cons of any and every drug should be considered. Another important example are the frequently used statin drugs that are known to deplete CoQ10.

There are two parts to the decisions you and your doctor make about medication. The first is which medication will be of greatest benefit to you in managing your glucose level without causing undue weight gain and complications. The second is how motivated you are to comply with instructions for defeating the roadblocks that can make you transition from prediabetes to type 2 diabetes. The decision of exactly how to treat your diabetes is often largely related to your willingness to make an honest agreement with your physician to make a very concerted effort to comply with that treatment.

KNOW WHICH MEDICATIONS ARE AVAILABLE

You are fortunate as a diabetic patient in the twenty-first century because you and your doctor have many more treatment options than ever before. Medical treatments for people with prediabetes and type 2 diabetes have evolved from the absence of any effective treatment in the nineteenth century to today's full range of drugs. Beginning with the development of a practical synthetic insulin in 1922, numerous targeted medications have become available to your physician. Prior to that date, diabetes was a certain death sentence. After 1922, oral agents to control blood sugar became widely available in the medications Micronase and Orinase. The medications you use can change over time because new, more effective glucose management techniques are emerging from breakthrough research. New drugs are rapidly appearing and might replace some medications that have been in use for decades.

The chart on page 65 lists medications developed by U.S. Department of Health & Human Services (July 1–2, 2008) and approved by the Food and Drug Administration (FDA) for prediabetes and type 2 diabetes. These medications are used singly and in combinations with other medications. Full descriptions of these medications and when and how they are used begins on page 67.

Classes of Drugs Approved for the Treatment of Type 2 Diabetes

DRUG CLASS	EXAMPLES	PRESUMED PRIMARY MECHANISM OF ACTION
Biguanides	Metformin (brand name Glucophage)	Decrease hepatic glucose production. Reduces liver insulin resistance
Thiazolidinediones	Pioglitazone (brand name Actos) Rosiglitazone (brand name Avandia)	Insulin sensitizers Modulate the transcription of genes involved in glucose metabolism
DPP-4 (dipeptidyl peptidase 4) inhibitors	Sitagliptin phosphate (brand name Januvia)	Slow inactivation of incretin hormones (e.g., GLP-1), which stimulate glucose-dependent insulin secretion
Incretin mimetics (glucagon-like peptide 1) analogues	Exenatide (brand name Byetta)	Stimulate glucose-dependent insulin secretion Promote satiety, increase glucose dependent insulin, slow stomach emptying Beta cell preservation
Sulfonylureas	Glipizide (brand name Glucotrol) Glyburide (brand names Micronase, Diabeta)	Stimulate insulin release by inhibiting the ATP-dependent potassium channel on pancreatic beta cells
Meglitinides	Nateglinide (brand name Starlix) Repaglinide (brand name Prandin)	Stimulate insulin release by inhibiting ATP-dependent potassium channels on pancreatic beta-cells (structurally different to sulfonylureas and exert effects via different receptors)
Alpha-glucosidase inhibitors	Acarbose (brand name Precose) Miglitol (brand name Glyset)	Delay glucose absorption from the gastrointestinal tract by inhibiting enzymes that convert carbohydrates into monosaccharides
Insulins	Rapid-acting, long-acting, mixed (brand names Lantus, Novolog, Humalog, Apirda, Levemir)	Stimulate peripheral glucose uptake by skeletal muscle and fat and inhibit hepatic glucose production
Amylin analogues	Pramlintide acetate (brand name Symlin)	Slow gastric emptying and suppress the postprandial rise in plasma glucagons Reduce hunger
Bile acid sequestrants	Colesevelam hydrochloride (brand name Welchol)	Reduce liver glucose May delay glucose absorption

In this chapter, you'll learn about the ability of these medications to control diabetes and why and when they are prescribed by your doctor. Some medications are prescribed only occasionally, such as the older sulfonylureas. Each year, newer and more frequently used drugs, such as Byetta and Januvia, come on the market and are quickly adopted because of their success. Despite how well they work for some people with diabetes who need to lose weight, medications are always used in the context of the patient's overall health condition.

The medications included in this step are considered the most effective of the drugs recommended for people with prediabetes and type 2 diabetes who must lose weight. (I regularly prescribe them in my practice.) Keep in mind that their effect on weight may be mitigated by their overall effect on your health if you do not take them as prescribed.

Breaking Roadblocks beyond Diabetes with Drugs

Modern drugs for prediabetes are effective for glucose and insulin management; they also help people to manage lipids and arteriosclerosis. For example, Actos slows the progression of arteriosclerosis and may possibly reverse it; Metformin and Byetta also reduce weight. But additional drug therapy will likely be necessary for continued obesity, hypertension, out-of-control lipids, fatigue, dysbiosis, and low hormone levels.

the hope study

One well-known drug study can give some hope to people with diabetes with cardiovascular complications.

The Heart Outcomes Prevention Evaluation (HOPE) study found that the ACE inhibitor ramipril (brand name Altace) can lower the risk of atherosclerotic disease events and death in patients without heart failure but with known atherosclerosis or with diabetes plus at least one cardiovascular risk factor. According to the study, "This benefit was independent of ramipril's effect on blood pressure. Additional benefits were a reduced risk of diabetic nephropathy in diabetic patients, and a lower likelihood of newly diagnosed diabetes. On the other hand, vitamin E in the doses and duration studied (400 IU/day for 4.5 years) did not lower risk significantly."

CONSIDER COMMONLY USED DIABETES MEDICATIONS
AND THEIR WEIGHT LOSS CONNECTION

All of the medications described below have specific goals: to regulate insulin supply through the pancreas, increase insulin sensitivity at the receptor sites, control elevated blood glucose, and preserve pancreatic beta cell function. This is a primary step to weight loss, and without this balance, you will not be able to lose weight as you adopt the other steps of this program. Whenever you're prescribed a new drug, ask why your physician has picked that specific medication.

The following information provides an overview and important information about the most frequently used medications for prediabetes and type 2 diabetes. Virtually all of them have side effects. Be aware that there is a difference between side effects, which can be expected and usually disappear or become manageable with time, and adverse effects, which might be life-threatening and could include allergic reactions, potential for overdose, and biological reactions such as fluid retention.

Like most medications, these drugs can interact with other drugs given for separate conditions.

A full description of the possible side effects, interactions, and adverse effects of all of these medications for diabetes, along with any other special warnings, are in Appendix 1, which begins on page 202. However if you suspect that your medications are not working properly, do not hesitate to contact your physician.

Biguanides

Overall, the biguanides, such as metformin (brand name Glucophage) are effective at controlling or regulating insulin levels released by the liver. They are sometimes called insulin-sensitizing drugs, helping to keep your glucose from fluctuating between meals. As a result, they are very effective at promoting weight loss. Their main action is to increase insulin sensitivity by making your insulin work better, lowering blood sugar, and keeping it moving properly in the bloodstream so it can be absorbed at the cellular level.

These drugs are commonly prescribed for prediabetes and type 2 diabetes. In the liver and in the peripheral muscles, they help insulin to work more efficiently. Thus, this medication blocks destructive biochemical pathways that enable high blood sugar levels to damage nerves and small blood vessels.

This class of drugs is available generically and is much less expensive than other medications. Among these drugs, metformin can prevent progression to type 2 diabetes.

The most common side effects of the biguanides are gastrointestinal. Glumetza and Fortamet are different versions of metformin that have fewer side effects. Gastrointestinal side effects seem to be decreased when Metformin is used with pioglitazone (brand name Actos) or sitagliptin phosphate (brand name Januvia).

Note: The source for all side effects and drug interactions for all drugs discussed in this chapter: www.drugs.com, used by permission.

Thiazolidinediones

TZDs or thiazolidinediones, such as pioglitazone (brand name Actos) and rosiglitazone (brand name Avandia), are another class of drugs that are widely prescribed. They help with lipid and triglyceride control, increase the body's insulin sensitivity, aid the storage of glucose in the liver, and preserve beta cell function.

Some controversy has been raised about one particular formulation of these drugs, rosiglitazone (brand name Avandia). While Avandia is still on the market, it has been identified as a drug that can increase the risk of cardiovascular events. In 2008 the American Diabetes Association advised against using Avandia.

This class of medication, however, is very effective in controlling diabetes because it helps preserve beta cell function and lowers insulin resistance.

Some sources report that thiazolidinediones might have no effect on weight loss or might even cause weight gain. But since they stabilize your glucose insulin levels, increase your metabolic rate, stop fatigue, and supply more energy so you can exercise more, you are more likely to sustain lifestyle changes.

Some studies claimed that this category of drugs hindered weight loss because it caused fluid retention, but other, more recent studies have refuted this claim and many physicians (including me) still use it frequently.

There has been evidence that weight gain is possible with Actos and it may have to be discontinued. This is less common when Actos is used in combination with metformin.

Actos has been proven in some studies to significantly improve insulin resistance and beta cell function.

The combination of a TZD medication and metformin can very effective.

New research shows it slows down arteriosclerosis, too.

You may also hear about this class of drug being combined with others. Two are Avandamet (metformin and Avandia or metformin and Actos) or Janumet (metformin and Januvia) or Avandaryl (Avandia and Glimipride).

Because of the controversy surrounding these drugs, make sure you fully discuss them with your doctor if they are suggested.

DPP-4 Inhibitors: A Breakthrough for Many with Prediabetes

The most common formulation for this medication is sitagliptin phosphate (brand name Januvia). It is one of a new class of medications to control blood sugar levels. It may be taken alone or with other medications and comes as a combination medication (with metformin) called Janumet.

Premarket studies of this class of drugs demonstrated that it was particularly effective when your body is not producing enough insulin or using it properly. Januvia has the ability to inhibit the DPP-4 enzyme, which results in better insulin action and increases your insulin levels at appropriate times. It also slows the deactivation of incretin hormones, (see page 70), also called GLP-1, which has a beneficial effect on blood sugar.

Januvia helps raise insulin levels, and it also lowers blood sugar before and between meals, and there is some evidence that it can decrease the amount of glucose that is created, but not to dangerous levels.

It is important to remember that DPP-4 inhibitors are generally most effective when combined with diet, exercise, and, possibly, other medications.

Studies showed improved blood sugar control when Januvia was used alone or with metformin, pioglitazone (brand name Actos), or rosiglitazone (brand name Avandia). Its effectiveness increases with diet and exercise to improve blood sugar levels in patients with both prediabetes and type 2 diabetes.

The most common side effects seen in Januvia's clinical studies were upper respiratory tract infection, sore throat, and diarrhea.

Incretin Mimetics: Are They Miracle Drugs?

One of the most promising and widely used classes of diabetes medications is exenatide (brand name Byetta), which came on the market in 2005. Byetta is the only brand name available so far, but this medication has been shown to be successful in helping control glucose in people with prediabetes, and it has been extensively tested in people with type 2 diabetes.

Incretins are hormones released by the gastrointestinal tract in response to food intake. They enhance insulin secretion, activate absorption, and maintain glucose metabolism. There is a good chance that with this drug, you will reduce or delay your chance of going onto insulin.

This type of medication is injected with a pen-like device, and most people adjust to using it fairly quickly. The pen provides a quicker mealtime insulin response than a slower acting pill. This drug regimen seems a much better choice than injecting insulin for achieving weight loss in type 2 diabetes because it affects insulin secretion at mealtimes, when you are most likely to add weight and your body detects a rise in blood sugar. It also slows the emptying of food from the stomach, making the brain think you are full.

Byetta must be taken 15 to 60 minutes before meals. You cannot take a dose and then skip the meal if you become busy; the Byetta will have no positive effect and you may then develop low blood sugar.

Byetta's basic function is to help your body control blood glucose levels by increasing the release of insulin from your pancreas, but in a more efficient

the latest approach to medication use: a new paradigm

Ralph A. Defronzo, M.D., in a landmark lecture at the 2008 American Diabetes Association Meeting, presented a new paradigm in the management of type 2 diabetes. After detailing the physiological problems of diabetes, he indicated the reason for his new program. His new research indicates that people with prediabetes have lost 50 percent of their beta cell function and people with type 2 diabetes at the time of diagnosis have lost 80 percent of their pancreatic beta cell function. Based on this, he proposed a three-part guideline for treatment to accomplish the following:

1. Prevent hyperglycemia (high blood sugar)
2. Reduce insulin resistance
3. Preserve beta cell function

To accomplish this, he proposed along with lifestyle changes a triple-drug therapy of metformin (Glucophage), a TZD (pioglitizone [brand name Actos]), and the incretin analog exenatide (brand name Byetta).

note: I have been using this triple-drug therapy for some time with my patients.

manner. This action also preserves beta cell function and slows progression from prediabetes to type 2 diabetes. Incretin mimetics often are used in combination with other medications (such as metformin [brand name Glucophage]) in patients with major weight problems, such as the morbidly obese, and in those for whom rapid weight loss is needed.

Some physicians believe the incretins are effective in helping people with prediabetes lose weight and in preventing the progression to diabetes and preserving pancreatic beta cell function. Studies have shown that people with high A1C blood levels will do as well with this medication as initial insulin therapy. Insulin and Byetta are comparable in their ability to reduce A1C levels, but Byetta is clearly superior to insulin in its weight loss effect. Studies show that when incretins are given with metformin, they lower the A1C by ½ to 1½ percent.

Sulfonylureas: An Older Class of Drugs, But Still Useful in Some Situations

The drugs glipizide (brand name Glucotrol), glyburide (brand names Micronase, Diabeta), glimepiride (brand name Amaryl), tolazamide (brand name Tolinase), and a few others are still prescribed, but they do not have the same long-term benefits as some newer drugs. They are seldom used, but nondiabetes specialists may prescribe them when better drugs are available. They are not recommended as a first-line medication and have no effect on weight loss.

This class of drugs was one of the first approved for diabetes, but they have fallen out of favor because of a reported link to increased incidence of heart disease, and because they may lead to beta cell burnout. They can increase insulin resistance by stimulating the release of too much insulin into your bloodstream. While they help control blood sugar, they are really less effective than newer drugs at treating the underlying pathology of diabetes.

Sulfonylureas have been on the market since 1955, and, as the first meds to actually lower blood sugar levels, they are responsible for saving many lives. Their effect is to increase the amount of insulin the body produces, but they are of limited usefulness for people with type 2 diabetes whose pancreas no longer produces beta cells. (Note: They have also been linked to increased risk for heart disease and beta cell burnout.) All the drugs in this class work in the same way to increase insulin and lower blood sugar released by the liver.

The drugs in this group came on the market at different times. The second-generation drugs such as glyburide (brand names Micronase, Diabeta) are considered superior because they are more effective in lowering blood sugar and also can be taken in smaller amounts.

Sulfonylureas have been reported to cause lowered blood sugar (hypoglycemia), especially during strenuous physical activity. The generics and brands such as glyburide (brand names Micronase, Diabeta) and glipizide (brand name Glucotrol) seem to reduce abrupt decreases in blood sugar and can reduce weight gain because they do their work quickly in the body.

Meglitinides: Drugs That Work Well in Combination

Meglitinides include repaglinide (brand name Prandin) and nateglinide (brand name Starlix), which came on the market between 1997 and 2000. They have the same basic effect as the sulfonylureas, but through a different mechanism. They bind to a different site on the beta cell called the ATP-dependent K+ (Katp) in a complex manner. These drugs are used infrequently today.

Taken before meals, these drugs stimulate insulin release from the pancreas if your blood sugar goes up after a meal, preventing a serious rise in blood sugar and acting in much the same manner as a healthy pancreas would. Their length of action is only two or three hours, so they provide an almost instant benefit, especially when taken shortly before meals. Consequently, this is a good medication for people with diabetes who have trouble reducing high carbohydrate use.

Taken alone or in combination with metformin (brand name Glucophage), these drugs also increase insulin at mealtime, but they do so abruptly. Thus, they're not particularly helpful with weight loss except in their ability to help reduce the negative effects of carbohydrates.

Repaglinide is used to treat type 2 diabetes, either alone or in combination with other antidiabetes medications, along with a diet and exercise program.

Alpha-Glucosidase Inhibitors: Weight Loss and Glucose Control

Unlike most diabetic medications, the alpha-glucosidase inhibitors such as acarbose (brand name Precose) and miglitol (brand name Glyset) prevent carbohydrates from being absorbed into the digestive tract, resulting in less glucose in the bloodstream, thereby contributing to weight loss.

This is good class of drugs, although they are not widely used. They can prevent progression from prediabetes to type 2 diabetes, but they never really caught on. Carbohydrate-blocking nutraceuticals (see Step Three) are used more frequently for this purpose and considered more effective.

These medications have many things going for them, nonetheless, especially for people with type 2 diabetes. While any medication that contributes to lowered glucose levels benefits weight loss, these drugs actually make weight loss less difficult. There is evidence that these can be used as a stand-alone or first-line medication in type 2 diabetes. These drugs are effective when taken with the sulfonylureas and metformin, and they are sometimes used with insulin.

The alpha-glucosidase inhibitors have some important dosing aspects. For example, they are literally supposed to be taken with the first bite of every meal. Their effectiveness is dose dependent, and it may take time for you and your doctor to adjust the dosage to get the desired effect. These medications are not recommended for people with kidney disease.

Do not take Precose when suffering diabetic ketoacidosis, which is a life-threatening medical emergency caused by insufficient insulin and marked by mental confusion, excessive thirst, nausea, vomiting, headache, fatigue, and a sweet, fruity smell to the breath.

You should not take Precose if you have cirrhosis (a chronic degenerative liver disease) inflammatory bowel disease, ulcers in the colon, intestinal obstruction or chronic intestinal disease associated with digestion, or any condition that could become worse as a result of gas in the intestine.

Special warnings about Precose: Every three months during your first year of treatment, your doctor will take a blood sample to determine how your liver is reacting to Precose. While you are taking Precose, you should check your blood and urine periodically for the presence of abnormal glucose levels.

Even people with well-controlled diabetes may find that stresses such as injury, infection, surgery, or fever can lead to uncontrolled blood sugar. If this happens to you, your doctor may recommend that Precose be discontinued temporarily and injected insulin used instead.

(See also Appendix 1.)

Insulin: Saving Lives Every Day

Brand names: Lantus, NovoLog, Humalog, Apidra, Levemir. There are three types of insulin: long acting, fast acting, and also mixed insulins, which are a combination of long and fast acting.

The first thing that may come to your mind about insulin is that you will be taking shots frequently during the day, like someone with type 1 diabetes (formerly known as juvenile diabetes). Insulin injections may make you may feel you've failed at controlling your disease, you may fear needles, or there may even be cultural or religious taboos. You might also worry that your job could be affected if it requires physical labor and your activities are restricted. Or you could just be embarrassed by being insulin-dependent. These are legitimate and common fears. But rarely does going on insulin make you feel worse, in fact, it helps you to feel better. You should not see taking insulin as a failure, but as a lifesaving drug that can be used after years of taking oral medication to keep you healthy.

Insulin can save your life, but it frequently causes weight gain because of its anti-lipolytic effect, which prevents fat from breaking down and promotes fat storage. Keep in mind that the healthier your lifestyle is, the less insulin you might need.

Insulin is a natural hormone generated in the pancreas. It is carried through the bloodstream to specific receptor sites that convey glucose into the cells, reducing the level of glucose in the blood. When this process gets out of whack, you are on your way to diabetes. If you load up with carbohydrates and other foods that raise your blood sugar, your glucose levels may even flood your urine and damage your kidneys, a condition called **glycosuria**.

The first reason you will need to inject insulin is that you have reached the "closed—too much glucose" sign at your receptor sites. If you aren't exercising or eating well and you are not burning off the glucose, your body begins to expel it from the kidneys in large amounts, and you may actually lose weight.

That's not good news in this case. When you inject insulin to get your body back on track, the pounds may quickly return. Why? You are still not exercising or eating properly. With insulin, your body's glucose levels generally will return to normal, and you can eat less and still have enough energy for exercise or simply to carry on daily activities.

Taking insulin is not a roadblock. How you take it, whether by a needle, a pump, or an injectible device like an EpiPen, does not matter. View it as simply another medication that can control your blood glucose levels. The common-sense aspects of a healthy diet and more active lifestyle—as you will learn in the next several steps—such as watching your caloric intake; learning the fundamentals of good nutrition; cooking healthy, low-fat meals; taking a walk instead of parking yourself in front of the TV; and so on, are designed to balance potential weight gain with drugs such as insulin.

As a type 2 diabetic who is dependent on insulin, it's always important to remember that you may have underlying conditions percolating, especially in your cardiovascular system—so keep your doctor informed if you are having any sort of reactions to your meds in general and insulin specifically.

Amylin Analogues

One medication, pramlintide acetate injection (brand name Symlin), often is prescribed along with insulin for certain patients (more likely type 1 but also sometimes type 2 diabetes) who have glucose fluctuations during the day. Used primarily before meals, this drug reduces blood sugar after you eat. There is some evidence that this medication, which is also taken by self-injection, may contribute to weight loss. Symlin is a synthetic version of a naturally occurring hormone, amlyn, that is produced by the beta cells, which also produce insulin in the pancreas.

MANAGE YOUR MEDICATIONS

The challenges of living with diabetes are unique, and one of the most important of these is the level of self-management required. In some ways, you become your own doctor, nurse, home-health aide, and nutritionist as you try to keep your blood sugars normal. In the past chapters, you've been told that you have to make dietary adjustments and add exercise and different drugs to a knowledge bank about diabetes and make some lifestyle adjustments. But there's more.

Your life-saving medications can become significant roadblocks to diabetic health—and especially weight loss—if you don't have and maintain complete control over them. Many people take multiple drugs, which complicates use and safety.

You might be taking many pills every day, giving yourself injections of one or two medications, and doing it in a order that keeps them working effectively. It's likely that you might take these medications for the rest of your life—or at least the near future—and as new ones come on the market, they may be substituted. In addition, you want to take nutraceuticals to assist you in weight loss.

The single most important aspect of managing your medications is ensuring that you are doing so safely. This means following instructions, learning about your medications, keeping your health-care team informed, watching for side effects, keeping careful track of them all, and taking your medications while traveling.

Following Instructions

Take medications exactly as prescribed unless your doctor tells you differently. Don't rely on a nurse, pharmacist, or other medical professional. Your doctor knows you best.

Do not stop taking a medication unless you are told to do so. Doing so can result in adverse effects on your heart or entire system.

Learning about Your Medications

It's not necessary to become a pharmacist, but you need to be as informed as possible about what you are taking. Learn all you can about the medications you are taking. Become an informed consumer.

Don't ever rely on what others such as relatives or neighbors tell you about your medications. Every medication today comes with a patient information sheet. Read it carefully, and if you don't understand it, ask your pharmacist and your doctor. Keep the patient information sheet in a file or somewhere handy for reference in an emergency.

Keep up with the news, new studies, and other reports on drugs. If you can, subscribe to a few online medical newsletters that can give you a good overview of the news and links to more reports in depth.

If you begin a new medication and develop side effects, call your doctor, talk to your pharmacist, or go to an emergency clinic if the side effects are severe or make you feel unusually ill. Describe your symptoms accurately and in detail.

It's important to read reports carefully to see whether they are based on a controlled study that matches the results of a real pill against a placebo. Some studies are meaningful; others may not really apply to you. Talk to your doctor about what you read in the newspaper.

Keeping Your Health-Care Team Informed

Tell all of your doctors what you are taking, especially when visiting a new doctor. Many people with diabetes go to a lot of doctors. Make sure you keep written records and let your doctor know what you are taking and about any changes in drugs or dosages.

Bring your drug record with you to each appointment.

After a while, you will learn to sense if a drugs is working so you can report this to your doctor. Ask your doctor when the medication should become effective. If you don't notice the prescription becoming effective within the specified time, call your doctor immediately.

Watching for Side Effects

Another important part of medication safety is being able to recognize side effects. Keep track of side effects and report them to your doctor—quickly—to see whether a different dosage or another drug will work for you. Note the difference between side effects, which are expected, and adverse reactions, which are unexpected and very serious. For example, a side effect might mean a stomachache or nausea, but an adverse effect might be severe swelling in your legs or severe shortness of breath.

If you experience an adverse reaction, call your doctor immediately or go to the emergency room.

Keeping Track of It All

This is key because a diabetic might require multiple medications and frequent doses, and forgetting a dose is not unusual. Here are ideas for getting and keeping a grip on it all:

- Develop a system for taking your medication. Some people keep their morning pills in one color of vial, their afternoon pills in another color, and their evening pills in a third.

- Ask your pharmacist to help you set up a system for keeping track of your medications. Pharmacists often have special labels or ideas about when and how you should take each pill.
- Buy pill holders that hold individual daily dosages for a one- or two-week period.
- Consider using pill cases with timers to remind you when to take your pills.
- Try to take your medication at specific times that will help you remember, such as before or after a meal.

Anything that makes compliance easier is worth trying.

Taking Your Medications While Traveling

Travel with medication can be complicated. Anyone who has flown anywhere within the past several years knows that you can take only certain things through security and in your carry-on luggage. Generally, you can pack any medication in checked luggage, but the risk of its being lost is not worth the convenience. You can carry medications you need on board with you, but take time before your flight to find out the current regulations for doing so. You can easily find these on the Transportation Safety Administration's web site: www.tsa.gov.

It's important to remember that medications are a key part of the solution. Medication—especially diabetes medication—is very effective in most cases. Taking more than one does not mean that you are failing, just that these ingredients in your program have to be assembled to fit your individual needs. New drugs appear constantly, and finding the right and best combo for you may take some time and changes.

Patience is essential to weight loss as a prediabetic or diabetic. Diabetes is yours forever, but it can be controlled. Your weight gain does not have to be forever. You may lose a significant amount of weight in the early stages of this program simply because your undetected or untreated condition has led to weight gain. Sooner or later, most people reach a weight loss plateau. As you get healthier, you will actually want your weight loss rate to slow somewhat, enabling your body to adjust to both your medications and the new nutritionally rich lifestyle you will learn about in Step Three.

Cutting Medication Costs

Prescription medications can be very expensive, and between 2001 and 2007, the cost of diabetes medications almost doubled. Too often, people face a terrible choice: Do I eat, get the pills, or buy gas to get to work? The pills may be the first thing to go. In addition, the cost of medications purchased under insurance plans may rise unexpectedly, along with your co-pays and deductibles.

Here are some ways to help keep medication costs down:

- Always ask if the medication is available in a comparable generic formulation.
- Visit websites that offer great ideas for saving on medication costs. We recommend this one, which lists more than seventy cost-cutting tips: http://yourtotalhealth.ivillage.com/medication-assistance-resources.print.html.
- Shop around. Many large retail operations, such as Wal-Mart, Target, and the "big box" clubs, offer hundreds of the most common medications, over-the-counter vitamins, and generic drugs for as low as $4 for a thirty-day supply. Several retail drugstore chains such as Walgreen's, have joined this trend. Check with your doctor about whether this option can work for you.
- Ask your doctor for samples when you start a new drug.
- Ask the pharmacist to only partially fill the prescription to make sure that you can tolerate it before wasting the money for a full prescription.
- Check with the drug companies for low-cost or free medications. Associations have been formed to offer this service, one of which is the Partnership for Prescription Assistance. Contact them at their website, www.pparx.com, or through your doctor. Dozens of pharmaceutical companies also offer these programs. Ask your doctor who makes your medications and go online to contact them or ask your doctor for the name of the drug rep for the medications.
- Older patients and people with limited incomes may qualify for special programs under Medicare Part D, Medicaid, or Social Security. Look into the coverage you have now and find out whether you can get additional help through supplemental programs, such as through the AARP.
- Check with your insurance company. For example, Medical Mutual has a program called Diabetes Advantage that provides insulin, a blood glucose monitor, test strips, needles, and sterile wipes at no cost. Each month, you speak with a nurse who keeps records of your progress and provides information when needed.
- Consider receiving your medications through mail-order discount drug programs such as www.medco.com and online services that provide meds in bulk at a very good discount, such as www.drugstore.com.

BECOMING A FAT-BURNING MACHINE!

Diet is, without a doubt, the keystone of diabetes control. A properly tailored diet holds your overall efforts together just as a keystone holds together an arch. Without the right diet, your medications won't work properly, and you won't have the energy to build muscle, be active, exercise regularly, and continue to lose weight.

In this chapter, you will learn how to overcome the food-based roadblocks to good diabetic health outlined in Step One by ensuring a sound diet and nutrition in your life. When you do this, you create catalysts for weight loss. Each change you make is a bio-trigger that alters your overweight body, transforming it from a fat-producing machine to a fat-burning engine.

Step Two has shown you how some roadblocks to weight loss are treated medically. The next task is to understand how important the foods you consume are—and how critical it is that they be matched to your specific needs. Your goal is to develop specific meal plans—not diets—that lead to glucose control and weight loss by helping you to make good food decisions. When you make these choices and are properly treated medically for prediabetes or type 2 diabetes and follow the steps outlined in Steps Four and Five, your success is guaranteed. All aspects of the program will act synergistically to achieve your goals.

Thousands of my patients at the Heart, Diabetes and Weight Loss Center of New York use the approach to weight loss explained in this step. Remember, this is a program to lose pounds and also to prevent life-threatening diabetic and cardio-vascular complications.

UNDERSTAND THE SPECIFIC BENEFITS FOR YOU IN THIS STEP

This program will help you to accomplish the following:

- Understand and enact the kind of diet that will most benefit you, if you have prediabetes or diabetes
- Gain the benefits of a complete nutritional evaluation
- Develop a meal plan designed to stop weight gain and reduce it through a balance of proteins and carbohydrates
- Eliminate adipose/visceral fat
- Control glucose and insulin levels
- Concentrate on a wide range of proteins
- Consume varied, moderate, low-carbohydrate meals
- Attain a correct level of carbohydrates starches in each meal (grams per day)
- Incorporate strong use of nutraceuticals (supplements and vitamins) to control appetite
- Feel satisfied/full without overeating or eating the wrong things
- Prevent bingeing and craving
- Enhance thermogenesis (fat-burning effect)
- Reduce inflammation (Inflammation is a silent killer and a component of every known degenerative disease, from heart disease to obesity.)
- Reduce beta cell stress syndrome
- Control gastrointestinal complications
- Reduce excess water in your body
- Avoid problematic food allergens
- Control carbohydrate addiction
- Learn the value of high-fiber foods
- Use foods with high nutrient density
- Achieve a marked reduction in simple sugars
- Identify low-glycemic foods
- Enjoy consuming unsaturated fats
- Eliminate trans fats

- Avoid artificial sweeteners
- Understand the caloric content of foods
- Make a sound meal plan and stick to it

This plan has been created to accommodate your real needs as a diabetic. The goals listed above will come about naturally as you make the right choices, based on real knowledge of your medical status, from the meal options at the end of this chapter.

You have probably heard of a "diabetes diet," often in negative terms. This is a tricky issue because on one hand, there is no single "diabetes diet," but on the other hand, there are dietary requirements for a diabetic. The diet you will eventually create here is designed to overcome the specific metabolic roadblocks you face. The proportions of carbohydrates and proteins vary in commercial diets, and while that may be fine for some people, for a diabetic, this combination has to be tailored to what your blood sugar levels are and whether you have concomitant disease. This plan also recognizes other dietary requirements you may have due to cardiovascular disease, which is common among people with diabetes.

STOP ON-AND-OFF DIETING

You probably know from hard and frustrating experience that changing your eating habits or lifestyle through a traditional diet is often a losing battle, not unlike climbing a mountain. While you seem to be burning fat for a while, you never quite fully succeed. Once you get close to the summit, you slide back down to your base camp, those old carbo-loading habits, and you are back to generating fat.

You may be stymied and frustrated because nothing seems to work. Depression and anxiety are common after attempts to lose weight fail.

Anyone who tells you that losing weight, especially while controlling one or two serious illnesses at the same time, is easy is being less than candid. If it were true, the medical problems of millions of obese people in this country would not be flooding the medical system. As I have already explained, the visceral fat that most obese people have as a result of genetics compounded by poor dietary choices and lack of exercise, is the hardest to lose. The truth is that you have a harder climb to successful weight loss than most overweight people without diabetes have. Losing weight for most people can be broken down to a few words: Burn more calories than you consume. It would be nice if this concept could apply equally and fully to people with prediabetes and type 2 diabetes, but a compromised metabolic state will usually defeat your efforts in the long run. Becoming a fat-burning machine is easy only when you are thin and in top shape.

To meet this challenge, you have to take control of your situation, especially where nutritional roadblocks are concerned. By following the complete process in these pages, you will eventually conquer the mountain, benefiting your physical and mental health. Successful weight management will not happen overnight, but this program will be safe, and it will prevent your prediabetes from progressing to type 2 diabetes or it will help you to control your blood glucose levels if you have diabetes. Always keep in mind that the goals are to be healthy, establish a better weight, prevent the loss of energy, and reduce the risks of blindness, kidney disease, amputation, and other complications.

At the beginning of this chapter, we told you that your diagnosis of prediabetes or diabetes was not your fault, that your genetics have likely sent you down this pathway. But when it comes to diet and nutrition, you can overcome the cards you were dealt. The only part that would be your fault is not trying to adopt a new healthy diet.

If your disease is not treated and your eating habits aren't modified, exercise won't help you very much. You might be too heavy to exercise enough to burn calories efficiently, you might have compromised joints or heart disease, or you might simply lack motivation or are depressed by your metabolic deficiencies. With this in mind, you cannot begin too soon to make good choices.

BEGIN SELECTIVE EATING

Can a food plan for people with prediabetes and diabetes really offer choices? Your bad choices led you to this point, and good choices will be the way you stop teetering on the edge of the health cliff. As you read through this step, you will see that there is very little magic. What you will find are *options*. Even if you are on medication for diabetes, you can select options that reduce the amount of medication you have to take.

The challenge you face is complicated because so much of the twenty-first-century American diet is processed food, high in sugar, chemicals, food additives, artificial sweets, trans fats, saturated fats, and calories. Your choices today are narrow, just as the aisles in the supermarkets are. To lose weight as a diabetic, you have to practice careful selective eating.

Here's what I mean. Most diets tell you to avoid foods such as meat and eggs, but for most people, including those with diabetes, lean meats, Canadian bacon, and eggs can be good sources of protein. You want to avoid foods that have highly saturated fats, such as fried foods. It does you no good where glucose control and weight loss are concerned if you deep fry your food. So selective eating enables you to eat foods you like—as you will see in the meal plans that begin on page 100—but not drenched in fat or cooked in a manner (such as fried) that negates the value of the food as part of a good nutritional program.

While this plan requires dedication and commitment, you will not have to adopt an extreme diet, depriving yourself of anything that tastes good and satisfies you. The secret is in the mix of elements, as you will see in the menus that follow.

The nutritional decisions that are suggested in this step do not begin with a list of foods or rules like other weight loss programs. This step begins with some nutrition related tests to supplement the general medical testing recommended and described earlier.

HAVE A BASELINE FOOD EXAM

Once your physician has completed the medical history, metabolic tests, and physical exam described in Step One, you should begin reviewing your nutritional profile—what you eat now—on your own or with a certified nutritionist, if possible. Most diabetic and cardiology specialists have a staff member (or department) who can help you understand why your current eating habits may be anchoring your weight.

The key tests like the A1C have already told you and your doctor if you have prediabetes or diabetes. Since the A1C test is done in the physician's office, the nutritionist will know where to begin, based on the level of glucose control you will need to establish through diet.

Just as the personal health questionnaire and the blood tests covered in Step One show where you are in need of help, the nutritionist can provide a picture of your eating habits and can help you take the next step to weight loss.

While most nutritional evaluations are really very simple, they should be as comprehensive and detailed as possible. You'll be asked to provide basic personal information, such as your weight, height, pulse, and blood pressure, and measurements of your waist, abdomen, chest, and hips.

The nutritionist will review with you how long you have been overweight and whether significant abdominal obesity is placing you at risk for cardiovascular disease. This is a crucial point for you. You must set aside any embarrassment and be honest with the nutritionist. Remember that the belly fat you're dealing with is not "subcutaneous fat tissue" under the skin, but fat deposits around your organs created by your insulin resistance.

In addition to establishing the metabolic parameters of your glucose, insulin, diabetic and prediabetic status; and your thyroid, hormone, and adrenal status; the nutritionist will use other instruments to check your metabolic rates, such as a body composition study, measurement of resting metabolic rate, and Heidelberg test.

Body composition study: One of these will be a body composition study, which is done to determine the exact proportion of lean body mass, including the percentage of muscle, body water, and fatty tissue. It also delineates the areas where there is most fat and calculates total percentage of body fat and body mass index (BMI—see page 88). This is extremely important as an initial evaluation to determine your exact body composition and to follow you as you lose weight to ensure that you are not losing lean muscle mass and to track tissue water loss.

Measurement of resting metabolic rate: You may also be asked to breathe into a device that measures your caloric/oxygen output. This tells you how many calories your body needs at rest and how many calories you will need to expend to lose weight. It measures resting energy expenditure/resting metabolic rate (REE/RMR), oxygen uptake, and calculates your BMI. It can be used to screen for slow metabolism and to construct a customized weight loss program. Periodic retesting will reveal the effect caloric reduction or medication is having on your metabolism. You will likely get a graph from this test that will help you gauge your current metabolic rate. The printed results are formatted to assist in *teaching energy balance* to patients in a colorful, easy to understand manner.

Heidelberg test: The third test, which is optional, is a Heidelberg test; it measures gastric acid. Many people have gastrointestinal problems that include lack of hydrochloric acid. The test measures hydrochloric acid and the patient's response to an alkaline agent to determine the degree of digestion. People who cannot properly digest food have problems with digestion and losing weight.

In addition to medications, supplements, and your general medical history, your nutritionist will focus on the following aspects of your nutritional habits:

- What you eat at breakfast, lunch, dinner, and as snacks
- Condiments you use
- Amounts and types of high-carbohydrate foods you eat
- Food allergies and sensitivities
- Amounts and types of fluids you drink, including alcohol

the body mass index (BMI)

According to virtually every authority, including the American Heart Association, "obesity" is "too much body fat." According to the National Heart, Lung, and Blood Institute, obesity is expressed in a ratio of your height and weight. This provides the Body Mass Index (BMI) value mentioned earlier, which is generally accepted as a measure of excess weight, if any, and the various health risks that follow.

Here's how to calculate your BMI: Multiply your weight (in pounds) x 704.5. Divide that number by your height (in inches), and then divide that number by your height again. Round up or down to the nearest whole number.

For example: 187 pounds x 704.5 = 13174.15. divided by 67 inches = 1966.29 divided again by 67 inches = 29.34. BMI equals 29.

note: This is a formula used by the National Institutes of Health (NIH). There is some small variation in the multipliers used by other groups; however, the difference is negligible.

Instead of doing this math, you can find your BMI on the chart on the follwing page.

- Digestive problems you have
- Gastrointestinal conditions, such as gas, bloating, indigestion, and constipation

The nutritionist might ask you to keep a daily diary of your current diet. While what you eat is important, equally important is how you eat. Do you respond to stress with a trip to the freezer to polish off the gallon of ice cream stashed there? Are you an emotional eater: Do you turn to food when you're happy, depressed, or excited? Are your meals at regular times, or do you find yourself eating dinner at 10:00 p.m. when you get home from work? Do you grab the first thing you come across because you're too tired to cook? Do your family's needs dictate when and what you eat?

Other aspects of a nutritional evaluation will include your level of physical activity, sleep patterns, occupation, stress level, how often you eat in restaurants and travel, ethnic food preferences, and any medications and nutritional supplements you take.

Interpreting Your BMI

If you have a BMI of 30 or above, you are technically obese. However, even if the number is below 30, you might not be in the clear. You still may be overweight. Multiple groups, such as the World Health Organization (WHO), define overweight as a BMI of 25 or higher. One of the problems with using the BMI scale is that many people who are fit and trim have a high BMI because their bodies are muscular. On the other hand, a person might have a low BMI, but be malnourished and unhealthy.

BMI is a good general measure because it is a simple reference point that you can use as a personal benchmark. The point is that if you have a high BMI, it is likely that you have a seriously increased risk for heart disease, high blood pressure, and diabetes.

body mass index table

for BMI greater than 35, go to Table 2

To use the table, find the appropriate height in the left-hand column labeled Height. Move across to a given weight (in pounds). The number at the top of the column is the BMI at that height and weight. Pounds have been rounded off.

BMI	19	20	21	22	23	24	25	26	27	28	29	30	31	32	33	34	35
Height (inches)	Body Weight (pounds)																
58	91	96	100	105	110	115	119	124	129	134	138	143	148	153	158	162	167
59	94	99	104	109	114	119	124	128	133	138	143	148	153	158	163	168	173
60	97	102	107	112	118	123	128	133	138	143	148	153	158	163	168	174	179
61	100	106	111	116	122	127	132	137	143	148	153	158	164	169	174	180	185
62	104	109	115	120	126	131	136	142	147	153	158	164	169	175	180	186	191
63	107	113	118	124	130	135	141	146	152	158	163	169	175	180	186	191	197
64	110	116	122	128	134	140	145	151	157	163	169	174	180	186	192	197	204
65	114	120	126	132	138	144	150	156	162	168	174	180	186	192	198	204	210
66	118	124	130	136	142	148	155	161	167	173	179	186	192	198	204	210	216
67	121	127	134	140	146	153	159	166	172	178	185	191	198	204	211	217	223
68	125	131	138	144	151	158	164	171	177	184	190	197	203	210	216	223	230
69	128	135	142	149	155	162	169	176	182	189	196	203	209	216	223	230	236
70	132	139	146	153	160	167	174	181	188	195	202	209	216	222	229	236	243
71	136	143	150	157	165	172	179	186	193	200	208	215	222	229	236	243	250
72	140	147	154	162	169	177	184	191	199	206	213	221	228	235	242	250	258
73	144	151	159	166	174	182	189	197	204	212	219	227	235	242	250	257	265
74	148	155	163	171	179	186	194	202	210	218	225	233	241	249	256	264	272
75	152	160	168	176	184	192	200	208	216	224	232	240	248	256	264	272	279
76	156	164	172	180	189	197	205	213	221	230	238	246	254	263	271	279	287

body mass index table (Cont.)

Table 2

To use the table, find the appropriate height in the left-hand column labeled Height. Move across to a given weight. The number at the top of the column is the BMI at that height and weight. Pounds have been rounded off.

BMI	36	37	38	39	40	41	42	43	44	45	46	47	48	49	50	51	52	53	54
Height (inches)	Body Weight (pounds)																		
58	172	177	181	186	191	196	201	205	210	215	220	224	229	234	239	244	248	253	258
59	178	183	188	193	198	203	208	212	217	222	227	232	237	242	247	252	257	262	267
60	184	189	194	199	204	209	215	220	225	230	235	240	245	250	255	261	266	271	276
61	190	195	201	206	211	217	222	227	232	238	243	248	254	259	264	269	275	280	285
62	196	202	207	213	218	224	229	235	240	246	251	256	262	267	273	278	284	289	295
63	203	208	214	220	225	231	237	242	248	254	259	265	270	278	282	287	293	299	304
64	209	215	221	227	232	238	244	250	256	262	267	273	279	285	291	296	302	308	314
65	216	222	228	234	240	246	252	258	264	270	276	282	288	294	300	306	312	318	324
66	223	229	235	241	247	253	260	266	272	278	284	291	297	303	309	315	322	328	334
67	230	236	242	249	255	261	268	274	280	287	293	299	306	312	319	325	331	338	344
68	236	243	249	256	262	269	276	282	289	295	302	308	315	322	328	335	341	348	354
69	243	250	257	263	270	277	284	291	297	304	311	318	324	331	338	345	351	358	365
70	250	257	264	271	278	285	292	299	306	313	320	327	334	341	348	355	362	369	376
71	257	265	272	279	286	293	301	308	315	322	329	338	343	351	358	365	372	379	386
72	265	272	279	287	294	302	309	316	324	331	338	346	353	361	368	375	383	390	397
73	272	280	288	295	302	310	318	325	333	340	348	355	363	371	378	386	393	401	408
74	280	287	295	303	311	319	326	334	342	350	358	365	373	381	389	396	404	412	420
75	287	295	303	311	319	327	335	343	351	359	367	375	383	391	399	407	415	423	431
76	295	304	312	320	328	336	344	353	361	369	377	385	394	402	410	418	426	435	443

LET'S GET STARTED NOW!

As the information below unfolds, you'll come to appreciate how understanding your roadblocks and making the dietary changes outlined here makes creating an effective meal plan easier.

As you change over to this meal plan, it is very important that you, your doctor, and your nutritionist meet to review the results of the tests outlined above and discuss your goals. Initially, the goals you set will not be about achieving a specific amount of weight loss. Instead your goal will be to ensure that the changes you make are in the context of your diabetes treatment and take into account any cardiovascular disease or high blood pressure that is present.

At the heart of the nutritional segment of the Five-Step Plan is the combination of carbohydrates and proteins you will choose, paying special attention to the amount and types of fat in your diet. How successfully you combine these elements depends upon your remembering that foods usually have more of one component than another. Vegetables, for example, are a combination of proteins and carbohydrates. The amount of each component in foods should guide your choice.

The Basic Food Types from a Diabetic Perspective

There is significant difference of opinion among nutrition experts, diabetologists, and cardiologists about the levels of carbs and proteins in the foods you should combine in your daily diet. Here are some basics facts to give you some perspective.

Carbohydrates are a primary component of starches, sugars, and even some fruits and vegetables. They are often referred to as "simple" sugars, "simple carbs," or "complex carbs."

The problem with controlling carbohydrates is that they dominate our meals today. There's the quick bagel at the train station as you rush to work, a sandwich at lunch, and starchy foods such as pizza at dinner. Carbohydrates of any kind have a positive primary role as a source of energy for our organs, cells, and tissues. We want carbohydrate-generated energy to circulate within our system, making us more alert, stronger, and able to exercise. Great athletes are known for carb-loading as they train to help them maintain a high energy level, and this is your goal, too. The problem is that you are not a world-class athlete training to run the marathon.

Here's where the story of the carbohydrates you consume is either good news or potentially bad news. Different types of carbs break down in the system more rapidly than others. Simple carbohydrates such as white or regular pasta, corn, sugared drinks, and juices are absorbed quickly and are transformed into glucose. That's great if your body is going to use them right away for fuel, but that's usually not the case in diabetics or obese people.

Complex carbohydrates, on the other hand, can be a good and valuable food because they break down more slowly in the bloodstream and they can add vitamins and minerals along with fiber to your nutritional needs. The simple carbs provide little nutritional advantage. Complex carbs include whole grain pastas and breads, brown rice, and other foods, some of which are listed later in this chapter.

Proteins, specialized molecules that help cells function, are often called the basic building blocks of our bodies. Insufficient protein intake compromises your body's ability to build muscle, produce red blood cells that increase oxygen levels in the bloodstream, increase muscle mass, strengthen cardiac muscle, and maintain organ function. The protein in your body is working pretty much all of the time.

The natural process of protein metabolism is the formation of amino acids. There is, however, one problem. Your body doesn't produce enough essential amino acids, so you need to eat more of foods that are rich in essential amino acids. Label reading and food charts will give you the information you need to find them.

Fat is found in most foods that are composed of fatty acids, which are essential components for blood clotting and maintaining blood pressure. There are three types of fats in foods: saturated fatty acids, polyunsaturated fatty acids, and monounsaturated fatty acids. Fatty acids are not in themselves good or bad. The important thing to understand when you are told to cut down on fatty foods is that you need to limit the amount and type of saturated fats you include in your diet. The secret is balance and moderation.

Generally, you'll find saturated fats in fatty beef, lamb, pork, butter, and shortening or oils derived from coconuts and vegetables such as peanuts. These fats are solid at room temperature. Saturated fats are converted by your liver to artery-blocking low-density lipoproteins ("bad" cholesterol). But some of these foods are also good sources of protein. The compromise is to limit the amount of these foods to a low percentage of your food intake.

A better choice is foods that contain polyunsaturated fats, which are liquid at room temperature. Corn, sunflower, soy, and cottonseed oils are generally high in polyunsaturated fats. Some fish have high levels of polyunsaturates and they may also have a good effect on your levels of high-density lipoproteins ("good" cholesterol). Still, be careful to limit the amount of these fats in your diet.

Foods or oils high in omega-3 fatty acids are mentioned frequently as a good source of nutrition and/or good for heart health. Omega-3 fatty acids are found in many fish, soybean and canola oils, and some nuts. Supplements of omega-3 fish oil are available in most drugstores and supermarkets. Many are coated for easy swallowing without the fishy aftertaste. Some heart patients take these daily.

Often called a "good" fat, monounsaturated fats are liquid at room temperature but may solidify in the refrigerator. These include olive and canola oils, many varieties of nuts, and avocados. Research shows that monounsaturated fats can help control "bad" cholesterol, but they may not necessarily decrease it. They make a good replacement for trans fats or saturated fats in your diet.

Trans-fatty acids have received a great deal of publicity recently. Essentially a blend of hydrogen molecules and vegetable oil, hydrogenated fats are found in cakes, cookies, fried foods, and products that need a longer shelf life. Hydrogenated shortening and oils should be avoided because they contribute to arterial blockage. Trans fats now have to be listed on the food labels of packaged goods.

How much fat should be in your diet? The answer to this is largely up to your doctor and your particular medical situation; however, federal government agencies such as the U.S. Department of Agriculture and the Department of Health and Human Services suggest that total fat intake should be limited to 35 percent of daily food consumption, and that this total should consist mainly of monounsaturated fats. Some extremely low-fat diets have reported success with a daily total fat consumption of 10 percent and complete avoidance of trans fats.

One last word about proteins, carbohydrates, and fats: In the real world, it is difficult to make a total change from one type of food to another. That's one reason this meal plan does not depend on counting calories, grams, or some other unit to gauge food choices, which is often an unrealistic and frustrating task. Steady dietary change and success in controlling your diabetes and dropping pounds help you to feel better, lose weight, and be excited about the changes in your body because you will like the new foods you eat.

Counting Calories

Think of a calorie as the amount of energy required to convert a certain amount of food to fuel. Calories are generally expressed in "units per gram." You might get 4 calories from a gram of carbohydrate or a gram of protein. When you consume high-calorie, fatty foods, and alcohol, more energy is released and more effort is required for you to use it up. If too many calories remain unused, those calories are stored as adipose tissue.

This weight loss approach does not put an emphasis on calories. While it is important to keep track of calories, properly balanced amounts of carbohydrates and proteins, combined with regular exercise, will help keep calorie intake under control. Your portion size, which should be normal, will also help control calories.–An excellent website to help you calculate calories is CalorieKing (www.calorieking.com), which has several different comprehensive lists and also free online calorie calculators.

CHANGE THE WAY YOU THINK ABOUT FOOD: THE WEIGHT LOSS BEGINS

Anyone who has ever tried to lose weight knows that the initial week or two is relatively easy, mostly because you may be losing fluids. But how do you change your eating habits so you're not tempted as you walk down aisles filled with cookies, candy, and cereals? For some people, just seeing the packaging can trigger strong desire.

There are real biological reasons why it is hard to resist the allure and fond memories of high-carbohydrate foods. As you eat these foods, chemicals called endorphins are released in your brain that carry signals to receptors in the pleasure center of your brain, increasing your desire for more of the same food. The pleasant feeling after eating foods high in sugar or starch—"comfort foods"— is caused by release of another chemical, serotonin, in the brain that produces a feeling of satiety or contentment.

Some scientists speculate that high-calorie, high-carbohydrate foods are also more likely to trigger compulsive eating because modern human beings evolved from primitive hunters who needed high loads of energy to survive. Over the centuries, we have sought these foods to stay alive. In effect, they became reinforcing, something that has stayed with us along with very little genetic change in the structure of our bodies.

One hundred years ago, the U.S. economy was still very much driven by physical labor. Daily survival was accomplished through hard work. We have the same biological needs today, but our way of life has become more sedentary, and "hunting" usually involves a short drive to a supermarket. There, we stalk our prey in a place so crowded with unhealthy, but convenient items that a biological disaster confronts us. If we get hungry, we don't need to make a spear and stalk four-legged food, we go to the refrigerator for food that will make us feel good and that is almost always available.

What happens biologically is that when we consume high-fat, high-carbohydrate food, the release of the chemical "reward" reinforces the feeling of pleasure associated with the food. This is where the real danger comes in. When you eat a food loaded with carbohydrates, your blood sugar shoots up, making you feel good and satisfied. But as soon as the carbs are absorbed, your blood sugar level drops, triggering the desire to regain the sensation of pleasure. So you head for more carbs. That is reinforcement. This creates adiposity and the potential for diabetes, heart disease, and stroke. You keep doing this because of the feeling of pleasure you receive, and it's more of a danger than a drug addiction because you must have food to survive.

OVERCOME SUPERMARKET ROADBLOCKS

One thing is certain: As you adopt a new approach to eating, you have to create a new approach to shopping for food. Supermarkets today can lure anyone, no matter how dedicated, to lose his or her way to good health.

Most people don't spend much time thinking about buying food that will help them overcome the unique biological challenge people with prediabetes and diabetes face daily. You have to do this now.

The desire for certain foods has been studied and reported on over the years. It's often been noted that people fantasize more about food than any other pleasure, including sex. After all, food gave us our first pleasure as children, and eating habits last a lifetime. Given the level of obesity in the country, is it any surprise that many adolescents who do their "hunting" in front of the computer or video game are following in their parents' footsteps?

Going to the supermarket is one of the few life-events we all share. After all, you have to get food somewhere, and for most of us, the supermarket or super-sized market is the primary option. Many of us enjoy going to the market. (Here's that silent reinforcement again.)

But for anyone with diabetes or weight problems, grocery shopping may be anxiety-producing, even a trap. But it doesn't have to be a negative experience, and you can turn it into a positive aspect of this Five-Step Plan.

Shopping Defensively

Here are some specific hints for defensive shopping:

- Prepare ahead. If there's one rule to follow, this is it: Don't to go to the supermarket "on the fly." We've all run out for a few things and ended up buying twice as much as we needed. Often, something in the store tempts us to do just that. For example, how many supermarkets position the bakery right where you walk in, with the wonderful smell of newly baked bread or cakes perfuming the air? It's not an accident.
- Consult your cookbooks and create a weekly menu. Write down all of the ingredients you need for it.
- Know what you are going to make, and make sure that most of what you buy fits into your overall meal plan.
- Check the fridge and pantry so you know what don't you need to buy.
- Shop weekly. Shopping too often or stretching your shopping trips to every two weeks will make sticking to your meal plan more difficult.
- Learn the store layout. The fewer tempting products you see and the less time you spend browsing, the easier it will be to avoid buying the wrong foods. The healthiest fresh foods are in areas against the store walls. Don't spend time in the central aisles with things you don't need.
- Look up and down. The most attractively packaged food is on shelves at eye level.
- Stay away from the areas where store employees are offering free samples of high-carb and fatty foods.
- Eat before you shop. A hungry shopper buys more food and makes worse food choices, plus with diabetes, you need to eat at specific times and in amounts that ensure stable blood sugar.

- Shop alone and without the kids. Although research claims that men are more likely to stick to their list only, the levels of obesity in both genders suggests otherwise. Going to the supermarket should be a directed, time-limited event. You are there to buy certain things you need; you don't have to review every single one of the store's offerings. If possible, shop for food when the kids are in school because they are special targets for marketers.
- Make healthy choices. This doesn't only mean buying fresh vegetables from local farms or good produce in the supermarket. A healthy choice is a meal you make at home—not take-out or prepared foods. Over the past decade, sales of prepared foods at the deli counters and throughout the store have risen steadily. Americans now spend over $15 billion per year on prepared foods in supermarkets and in shopping mall food courts.

While sales of starchy, fat-dripping fast foods are dropping, prepared take-out foods aren't much better. The choices are often "family friendly": fried chicken, chicken nuggets, chicken wings, baked potatoes, egg rolls, tacos, and creamy "comfort food" soups. Did you know that much of the prepared supermarket food is made by the same giant food companies that make the fast foods? If you buy prepared foods, avoid those with heavy mayonnaise or breading and high calories. Dodge items featuring rice or mashed potatoes, too.

Some experts suggest you take a close look at how much of your diet comes from the prepared choices. If prepared food makes up more than half of your diet, you have a problem. While one solution would be to learn to cook more or better, some people simply don't like to cook or have too little time to make meals at home. But this isn't an insurmountable problem.

Making the Supermarket Your Support System

If you are truly going to make a change that will bring your glucose under control and help you lose weight, you will have to take control of what you and your family eat. It is less difficult than you think. The secret is in your commitment to change.

There are scores of healthy-eating-oriented cookbooks in bookstores, supermarkets, mega-stores, and online recipe sources. These books help you follow some basic rules that will help meet the requirements of the Five-Step Plan.

Doing your own cooking will help you control what you eat, control your glucose, and lose weight. You will still go to the supermarket, but buying fresh vegetables in season, certain fruits, and good protein sources such as fish, chicken, turkey, and other lean meats will make your diet more interesting and flavorful. You might even discover that cooking can be fun, and you can make it a group activity. As you lose weight, you will feel better physically and mentally because the food you eat will be better for you. Your body will thank you.

Another good tip is to ask questions at the market. You'd be surprised how much help the people behind the counters can be, and not only at high-end supermarkets.

LEARN THE FIVE-STEP WEIGHT LOSS APPROACH

This weight loss approach combines the lessons of various approaches to weight loss for people with diabetes that we have learned from clinical experience, so you are more likely to stick with it. This diet will be easier than other diets to integrate into your daily life because it gives you choices.

This plan is essentially a combination of low-glycemic foods, reduced carbohydrates, and a modified Mediterranean diet. It is based on healthy proteins, minimal amounts of unsaturated fats, and use of monounsaturated fats, fiber, salad, vegetables, some nuts and seeds, whole grains, olive oil, and limited red wine. The carbohydrate content depends on your level of risk as indicated by your blood glucose levels.

In general, the initial program for people with higher glucose, A1C levels, and obesity allows approximately 45 grams of carbohydrates per day, spread between two or three meals: 15 grams at each meal to begin with for those with high risk of developing diabetes or who have very high blood glucose and A1C readings.

As you start to lose weight and your glucose level decreases, you will be able to increase the amount of carbohydrates you consume. For example, if your A1C is well below 7, you will be able to increase carbs slowly. The meal plan does not expect you to count carbs, but the plan and the menus will put you within those guidelines. Bear in mind that this low-carb plan involves minimal amounts of fruit and no fruit juices. (You eat fruits such apples, pears, oranges, and grapefruit.)

Are desserts are a thing of the past? In general, desserts are not allowed initially for people with high A1C who are not able to lose weight. However, as your hemoglobin A1C falls below 7 and with a limited amount of protein, fat,

diabetes food Q&A

Here are a couple of common questions.

Can you drink if you have diabetes? Multiple studies have been conducted on drinking and alcohol, and most indicate that "moderate" drinking is not harmful—depending on your gender. In fact, a group from the Nurses Health Study, one of the longest running health studies in the United States, was initiated in 1976 with a goal to evaluate factors that contribute to disease—especially cancer—among women. The program grew and eventually 238,000 nurse-participants provided "landmark" data on general female health and specific information on cardiovascular disease, diabetes, and lifestyle factors that influence disease. The Nurses Study indicated that for women "moderate drinking may be associated with a lower BMI." Moderate drinking is usually defined as no more than one alcoholic drink or two glasses of wine a day. Just remember that alcohol is very fattening and in the strictest weight loss programs no alcohol is allowed for either men or women. In more moderate plans, one alcoholic beverage may be allowed.

Do you benefit from eating slowly? While there are not many studies, eating slowly has proven to be an aid in weight loss. Eating until full ("I'm stuffed") or eating fast has a direct relationship to increased risk of weight gain. In fact it triples the risk. If you eat slowly, you savor your food more and are less likely to overeat. Train yourself to eat a meal only until you feel satisfied. Keep in mind that horrible feeling you have when you overeat.

and salad. An occasional dessert will be acceptable because eating a high-carb dessert with a protein helps slow absorption of the sugar.

In this meal plan, you can change the food options significantly as long as you select an appropriate ratio of carbohydrates to proteins. The food lists that follow at the end of this section will show you how to choose foods that appeal to you and that maintain this ratio.

Recent studies show that when the ratio of carbohydrates to proteins is kept low, the fat-reducing equation is at its most effective level. For that reason, when you choose from the lists that follow, reduce the amount of starch (such as bread, certain pastas, rice, potatoes, cereals, and fruit juices) and select salads, veggies, and protein.

I suggest the following diet/weight for people who are newly diagnosed with either prediabetes or type 2 diabetes. It gives you an entire week of meals to get you on your way to weight loss and put healthy food on your table.

Here are a few general guidelines to follow:

- In general, in the menus that follow, you want to combine a vegetable, a protein source, and an equal or lesser amount of a carbohydrate source.

- With regard to portion size, be sensible. A visual guide to portion size is to consider a standard-size (8-inch [20 cm]) plate as your meal size. Visually divide it into thirds, with each section filled (not over-filled) with one carb, one protein, and vegetables. If you leave the table feeling stuffed, your portions are too large.

- I recommend limiting or even omitting wheat products altogether. Wheat is a very common allergen that in my experience is a major block to weight loss. In addition, wheat and its proteins, gluten and gliadin, are highly inflammatory, causing tissue damage and immune challenges and further contributing to weight struggles. Instead, I suggest eating wheat free/gluten free breads or breads low in wheat such as brown rice bread, kamut bread, spelt bread, sprouted whole wheat bread, rye bread, or pumpernickel bread preferably from health-food stores, not supermarket breads. Wheat is found in all products made from flour, such as breads, bagels, muffins, pasta, cakes, cookies, pastries, and pies, and it is also found in many sauces along with cornstarch for its thickening properties.

- I highly encourage my patients to have a nice, large, green salad for lunch and dinner—preferably not made from iceberg lettuce. Eating a salad prior to meals helps to fill us up and slows down our eating so we eat less of the main meal. I highly recommend using natural dressings of extra virgin olive oil and vinegar or lemon, as the oils found in commercial dressings are toxic and detrimental to our health. In addition, most dressings contain MSG, which encourages us to eat more and store more fat.

A week of meals

MONDAY	TUESDAY	WEDNESDAY	THURSDAY
Breakfast	**Breakfast**	**Breakfast**	**Breakfast**
1 hard-boiled egg and 1 or 2 egg whites ½ grapefruit Coffee or tea, without sugar or artificial sweetener	Egg omelet of 2 or 3 egg whites and 1 whole egg, plus low-fat ham, low-fat cheese, and green pepper Coffee or tea, without sugar or artificial sweetener	3 ounces (85 g) of either Canadian bacon or turkey sausage, trimmed of fat One slice low-carb, whole grain, non-wheat bread, toasted Coffee or tea, without sugar or artificial sweetener	Scrambled eggs made with 1 whole egg and 2 egg whites Turkey sausage ½ grapefruit Coffee or tea, without sugar or artificial sweetener
Lunch	**Lunch**	**Lunch**	**Lunch**
Salad of lettuce, tomatoes, and cucumber Turkey or chicken breast, without skin	Tuna salad with light mayo, lettuce, celery, and olives	Salad of lettuce, tomato, and cucumber Low-fat ham Low-fat cheese	Salad of lettuce, tomato, green peppers, and olives Tuna or salmon salad with light mayo
Dinner	**Dinner**	**Dinner**	**Dinner**
Salad of lettuce, tomatoes, and cucumber Grilled or steamed fish, lobster, or shrimp 1 or 2 servings of green beans, asparagus, or cauliflower One slice low-carb, whole grain, non-wheat bread	Roast lamb, veal, or lean pork, without fat Salad of lettuce, tomato, and radish Broccoli and cauliflower One slice of low-carb, whole grain, non-wheat bread	Grilled or steamed fish, lobster, or shrimp Green beans, spinach, or asparagus Apple for dessert	Grilled white meat chicken, without skin Carrots, green beans, or spinach One slice low-carb, whole grain, non-wheat bread

FRIDAY	SATURDAY	SUNDAY
Breakfast	**Breakfast**	**Breakfast**
½ cup oat bran with a small amount of skim milk Apple or pear Coffee or tea, without sugar or artificial sweetener	Omelet made of 1 whole egg, 2 or 3 egg whites, low-fat cheese, green peppers, mushrooms, and 3 ounces (85 g) of either turkey or Canadian bacon Coffee or tea, without sugar or artificial sweetener	½ grapefruit One slice low-carb, whole grain, non-wheat bread Coffee or tea, without sugar or artificial sweetener
Lunch	**Lunch**	**Lunch**
Raw vegetables or large salad Turkey, chicken, or low-fat ham	Grilled white meat chicken or turkey burger Raw carrots, broccoli, peppers, and celery or cauliflower	Tuna or salmon salad with light mayo Salad of lettuce, tomato, cucumber, green pepper, and radish
Dinner	**Dinner**	**Dinner**
Chopped lean ground sirloin, grilled Salad of lettuce, tomato, and celery One slice low-carb, whole grain, non-wheat bread Brussels sprouts, asparagus, or green beans	Fish, lobster, or shrimp Salad of lettuce, tomato, celery, and radish Steamed or raw broccoli and cauliflower One slice low-carb, whole grain, non-wheat bread	3 ounces (85 g) filet mignon or lean steak, fat trimmed Steamed, grilled, or raw broccoli, cauliflower, asparagus, or green beans

A Month of Menus

Now that you are on your way to putting good healthy choices in front of you and your family at mealtimes, here's a month-long list of menus. Each meal gives you several different options to choose from. This dietary option plan will help you adjust to the kinds of foods that will encourage your body to use the

	BREAKFAST	LUNCH
wk1	Two scrambled eggs with Canadian bacon or turkey sausage	Prior to lunch, have a large green salad, preferably not iceberg lettuce, with a small amount of sugar-free prepared dressing or olive oil and vinegar. Eat salad before starting the main course.
	1 slice rye toast, with butter	One serving of carbohydrate can be chosen for lunch: 1 slice of wheat-free bread; ½ cup (80 g) brown or wild rice; ½ cup (70 g) of peas, beans, or chickpeas; ½ cup (90 g) lentils; or half of a small baked sweet potato. Choose one lunch of the following.
	3 ounces (85 g) Swiss cheese, 1 slice of tomato, and 1 slice of rye toast	
	Sliced Nova (lox) with 1 tablespoon (16 g) of cream cheese on 1 slice of pumpernickel	Broiled chicken with sautéed broccoli
	Two eggs sunny side up, with 2 slices of Canadian bacon, and 1 slice of spelt bread	Grilled shrimp with lemon, without catsup, with green salad or vegetables
	4 ounces (114 g) regular cottage cheese with ½ cup (80 g) cantaloupe or berries (65 g)	Can of wild salmon with half avocado over a bed of mixed greens
	1 tablespoon (16 g) almond nut butter with 1 slice of avocado on 1 slice of spelt bread	Scoop of chicken salad with light mayonnaise, beet salad, and steamed asparagus
	3 ounces (85 g) halibut salad with light mayonnaise on 1 slice of rye bread	Mixed green salad with goat cheese, chickpeas, walnuts, and half diced apple
	Western omelet made with egg whites, low-fat ham, green peppers, onion, and mushrooms	Broiled burger, without bun or catsup, with steamed broccoli or mixed green salad
		Caesar salad with chicken or shrimp, without croutons, with dressing on the side

protein and carbohydrates in the healthiest manner. Using a meal plan like this is an important aspect of losing weight and controlling your blood sugar levels at the same time.

The following menus contain common foods that you can choose from for different meals, or you can substitute one for the other.

SNACK	DINNER
This is a great snack to have each afternoon. Ten raw or dry roasted almonds and one small apple	Dinner is an important meal, and it should be comprised of ⅓ carbs, ⅓ proteins, and ⅓ vegetables. Prior to dinner, have a large salad with a small amount of sugar-free prepared dressing or olive oil and vinegar. Eat salad before starting the main course. Here is a partial list of some of some good carbohydrate choices to include in your dinners. (Note: net carbohydrates means total carbohydrates minus the carbohydrates in the products that don't affect blood sugar, such as fiber or sugar alcohols.) 3.5 ounces (100 g) baked sweet potato: 21 grams of carbohydrates 3.5 ounces (100 g) russet baked potato: 22 grams of carbohydrates 4 ounces (114 g) brown or wild rice: 23 grams of carbohydrates 4 ounces (114 g) cooked quinoa: 33 grams of carbohydrates 4 ounces (114 g) cooked lentils: 20 grams of net carbohydrates 4 ounces (114 g) cooked white beans: 22 grams of net carbohydrates 4 ounces (114 g) cooked red beans: 12 grams of net carbohydrates 4 ounces (114 g) cooked corn: 15 grams of carbohydrates 1 medium size corn on the cob: 15 to 20 grams of carbohydrates 1 slice of whole grain bread: 15 grams of carbohydrates 3.5 ounces (100 g) cooked spaghetti: 26 grams of net carbohydrates 3.5 ounces (100 g) whole wheat spaghetti: 22 grams of net carbohydrates For your dinners, the protein and vegetables are totally up to you. There are thousands of different foods out there, but many are extremely unhealthy. You have to look for very healthy choices like these. Broiled lamb chops, sautéed escarole, and 3.5 ounces (100 g) baked Russet potato Broiled wild salmon with dill sauce, sautéed kale, and ½ cup (90 g) cooked quinoa Broiled filet of sole with lemon and white wine, 3.5 ounces (100 g) baked sweet potato, and sautéed asparagus Broiled steak of choice (lean cut), steamed broccoli, and ½ cup (80 g) cooked brown rice Meatloaf, sautéed snap peas, carrots, celery, Shiitake mushrooms, and ½ cup (80 g) cooked wild rice Grilled shrimp and scallops, sautéed broccoli, and ½ cup (80 g) brown or wild rice Broiled pork chop (center cut, lean, trimmed), beet salad, sautéed kale, and 3.5 ounces (100 g) baked Russet potato

	BREAKFAST	LUNCH
wk2	2 ounces (57 g) fresh mozzarella cheese, melted on 1 slice of whole grain wheat-free bread	Turkey burger, without bun or catsup, with mustard and sautéed broccoli
	1 tablespoon (16 g) cashew nut spread and 1 slice of avocado, on 1 slice of rye bread	Broiled pork chop (center cut, no fat) with spinach salad
	Scrambled eggs with cut-up vegetables, with 1 slice of buttered spelt bread	Chili with meat and sautéed broccoli or mixed green salad
	4 ounces (114 g) regular ricotta cheese sprinkled with cinnamon on 1 slice of pumpernickel	Scoop of chicken salad with light mayonnaise on a plate of mixed greens
	3 ounces (85 g) sliced natural turkey breast with mustard on 1 slice of rye bread	Baked salmon with Dijon mustard with steamed asparagus or salad
	Western omelet, slice of cheese, with 1 slice of pumpernickel bread	Regular cottage or farmer cheese with berries and 15 almonds
	Scoop of chicken salad with light mayonnaise on 1 slice of spelt bread	Scoop of halibut salad with light mayonnaise on a spinach salad
wk3	1 tablespoon (16 g) organic peanut butter with sliced avocado on 1 slice of rye bread	Roast chicken with spinach salad or steamed asparagus
	3 ounces (85 g) goat cheese on 1 slice of pumpernickel and celery sticks	Grilled shrimp and scallops on a bed of mixed greens
	2 hard-boiled eggs with 1 teaspoon of light mayonnaise and 1 slice of rye toast	Lean beef burger, without bun or catsup, with onions, tomato, and side of vegetables
	Sliced turkey breast with mustard on 1 slice of brown rice bread	Scoop of egg salad with light mayonnaise on a bed of mixed greens
	Sliced Nova (lox) with cream cheese on 1 slice of pumpernickel	Lamb/beef/chicken kebab with mixed green salad or vegetables, without pita or other breads
	2 eggs sunny side with 1 slice of cheese and 1 slice of spelt bread	Whole grain taco with chopped meat, yogurt sauce, cheese, lettuce, tomatoes, and vegetables
	Nitrate/nitrite-free turkey sausage with two scrambled eggs and ½ grapefruit	Omelet with vegetables (peppers, onions, etc.) with beet salad or cole slaw
wk4	Sliced Nova (lox) with cream cheese or avocado on 1 slice of rye bread	Grilled shrimp over a mixed green salad with olive oil and vinegar or lemon
	Scoop of farmer cheese with sprinkled cinnamon on 1 slice of sprouted bread	Scoop of chicken salad with light mayonnaise with green salad or leftover vegetables
	1 tablespoon (16 g) almond nut butter with sliced avocado on 1 slice of pumpernickel bread	Broiled bison burger, without bun or catsup, with steamed asparagus and beet salad
	2 scrambled eggs with Canadian bacon and 1 slice of rye toast	Scoop of cottage cheese with melon and berries and 10 to 15 almonds
	Scoop of halibut salad with light mayonnaise on 1 slice of sprouted wheat bread	Chicken kebab with mixed green salad or sautéed eggplant and garlic
	Sliced turkey breast and Cheddar cheese with mustard on 1 slice of rye bread	Can of wild salmon with avocado and tomato on a bed of mixed greens
	Western omelet with nitrite/nitrate-free breakfast sausage and 1 slice of rye toast	Chili made with chopped, sautéed turkey meat and spinach with olive oil and garlic

SNACK	DINNER
Afternoon Snack: 1 tablespoon (16 g) either natural peanut, almond, or cashew butter on 2 large celery sticks Evening Snack: 3 ounces (85 g) plain, regular cottage cheese sprinkled with cinnamon	Baked or broiled flounder with lemon and white wine, sautéed asparagus, and 3.5 ounces (100 g) baked sweet potato Homemade chicken soup with lots of fresh or frozen vegetables and ½ cup (80 g) brown rice Nitrate/nitrite-free sausage and peppers, beet salad, ½ cup (70 g) pasta and steamed asparagus Broiled codfish with lemon and white wine, sautéed spinach, and ½ cup (80 g) wild rice Broiled chicken with lemon and rosemary, sautéed broccoli rabe, and 3.5 ounces (100 g) baked Russet potato 3 ounces (85 g) broiled or grilled filet mignon, steamed broccoli, fennel salad, and 3.5 ounces (100 g) baked sweet potato Sautéed chopped turkey meat with onions, peppers, and sautéed cabbage and ½ cup (80 g) brown rice
Afternoon Snack: 10 walnuts Evening Snack: 2 ounces (57 g) Swiss cheese with celery sticks	Broiled chicken, sautéed string beans, and ½ cup (80 g) brown rice Baked codfish, sautéed broccoli and carrots, and 3.5 ounces (100 g) of baked Russet potato Broiled lamb chops, steamed asparagus, and 1/2 cup (90 g) of cooked lentils Sautéed chopped meat with onions, peppers, carrots, and celery; large salad; and 3.5 ounces (100 g) Russet baked potato Broiled trout or Bronzini fillet, sautéed broccoli, and 3.5 ounces (100 g) of baked sweet potato Broiled veal chop, beet salad, steamed cauliflower, and 1/2 cup (80 g) of wild rice Sautéed shrimp, scallops, carrots, mushrooms, celery, and onions with ½ cup (80 g) of brown rice
Afternoon Snack: 2 ounces (57 g) Cheddar cheese with celery sticks Evening Snack: 1 tablespoon (16 g) plain, regular cream cheese with celery sticks	Broiled filet mignon, steamed broccoli, and 3.5 ounces (100 g) baked sweet potato Broiled wild salmon, sautéed bok choy, and ½ cup (80 g) brown rice Baked chicken (any part), steamed asparagus, and 3.5 ounces (100 g) baked Russet potato Broiled pork chop, beet salad, spinach salad, and ½ cup (90 g) quinoa Broiled filet of sole with lemon and white wine, sautéed broccoli, and ½ cup (80 g) wild rice Sautéed chopped turkey meat, onions, celery, carrots, and snap peas; green salad; and 3.5 ounces (100 g) baked sweet potato Steamed, grilled, broiled, or sautéed lobster and shrimp or seafood platter; broccoli, string beans, or salad of choice, and 1/2 cup (100 g) of potato salad or 3.5 ounces (100 g) of baked potato

ASSEMBLE YOUR WELL-STOCKED DIABETIC PANTRY

People with diabetes should have certain things in their pantries that they can reach for when an unexpected guest appears or you may have failed to plan for today's lunch or dinner. This doesn't mean that this is all you need to have in your kitchen cupboards, but to stay with the eating plans in this step now is the time to overhaul your pantry. You need to eliminate some foods. Take frosted cereals, pastries, and sugary candies off the shelves. Replace fruit punches and cocktail mix, regular soft drinks, and other sugary beverages with water and seltzers.

Common Carbohydrate-Rich Foods

Food	15 Grams of Carbohydrate per Serving
Apple	Small (size of tennis ball)
Beans	½ cup (100 g)
Brown rice	⅓ cup (53 g)
Cooked vegetables	1½ cups (approximately 150 g)
Orange	Small (size of tennis ball)
Raw vegetables	3 cups (approximately 240 g)
Rice cakes	2 regular cakes
Saltine crackers	6
White pasta, cooked	⅓ cup (50 g)
White rice, cooked	⅓ cup (53 g)
Whole grain pasta, cooked	⅓ cup (50 g)

A carbohydrate is a carbohydrate is a carbohydrate. All carbohydrates have an effect on your blood sugar. Be aware when reading labels. The words carbohydrate, complex carbohydrate, sugar, sugar alcohol, high fructose corn syrup, and even fiber refer to carbohydrates.

Market twice a week for fresh diary products, fish, meat, poultry, and produce and prepare the daily recipes using the staples in your pantry. Keep your pantry inventory turning. Things bought in too large a quantity can become rancid. Spices lose their aroma and flavor, and oil loses its freshness.

Stocking Your Cupboard

Standard baking needs as called for in the recipes.

Beans and Legumes (limited because of high carbohydrate content)

Black-eyed peas

Cannellini

Chick peas

Lentils, brown and
   red

Navy beans

Pinto beans

White beans

Dried Herbs and Spices

Allspice

Basil

Bay leaves

Caraway seed

Celery seed

Chili powder

Cloves

Coriander

Cumin

Curry powder

Crushed red pepper

Dry mustard

Fennel seed

Fine herbs

Ginger

Marjoram

Paprika

Peppercorns

Poppy seeds

Rosemary

Sage

Saffron

Savory

Sesame seeds

Thyme

Stocking Your Freezer

Bread dough, whole
   wheat

Breads and rolls,
   multigrain

Butter, unsalted

Fruits and berries,
   frozen, no-sugar-
   added

Nuts

Pita

Vegetables, steam-
   able in bags

Stocking Your Refrigerator

Anchovy paste in the
   tube

Butter, unsalted

Cheese, low-fat cream

Cheese, low-fat
   mozzarella

Cheese, whole-milk
   parmesan

Dill pickles

Eggs

Fruit, fresh apples,
   lemons, limes,
   pears

Ginger

Herbs, fresh

Milk, skim

Parsley

Pesto paste in the
   tube

Tomato paste in the
   tube

Vegetables, fresh
   and in season

Stocking Up on Meats

Store these in your refrigerator or freezer. All should be lean.

Beef

Cube steak, trimmed

Flank steak, lean, trimmed

Ground beef, 95 percent lean/5 percent fat

New York steak, trimmed

Porterhouse steak, trimmed

Round or loin cuts, with all visible fat trimmed

Round steak or roast, trimmed

Sirloin, trimmed

Strip steak, trimmed

T-bone steak, trimmed

Tenderloin (filet mignon), trimmed

Pork

Canadian bacon

Center loin, trimmed

Ham, lean, trimmed

Lean cuts, trimmed

Leg, trimmed

Loin, trimmed

Sirloin, trimmed

Tenderloin, trimmed

Top loin

Lamb

Leg, trimmed

Loin, trimmed

Poultry

Chicken breast and other white meat, without the skin

Chicken, broiler or fryer, lean meat only

Chicken, canned*

Chicken, dark meat without the skin

Chicken, ground

Chicken, roasted

Cornish hen, without the skin

Duck, domestic, without skin (Domestic duck is healthier and contains fewer chemicals.)

Turkey, canned*

Turkey, dark meat, without the skin

Turkey, ground

Turkey, white meat, without skin

*Canned meats do not need refrigeration until after opening.

Starches and Grains (use sparingly)

Barley	Kasha (buckwheat	Rice, brown
Bran, no sugar added	groats)	Rice, wild (use
Buckwheat	Millet	sparingly)
Bulgur	Quinoa	Rolled oats (Irish
Couscous, whole wheat	Pasta, whole wheat	oatmeal)

Potatoes (use sparingly)

Baby	New	Sweet
Bliss	Red	White

SUPPLEMENT YOUR DIET WITH NUTRACEUTICALS

My patients with diabetes often ask me about supplements. This interest has increased the use of supplements in the program. A considerable body of research shows the positive results of supplements, vitamins, and minerals in the enhancement of overall health. In fact, it's becoming clear that vitamins and minerals are effective co-factors for both insulin and glucose regulation. Many nutrients are also helpful in weight loss and fat control, as we shall see in this following section.

Anyone who has been in a pharmacy, health-food store, supermarket, superstore, or mini-mart knows that vitamins, supplements, and other nutraceutical products are widely available. Your pediatrician likely has urged you to give

A National Responsibility

The goal of this third step is not simply to help you lose weight with the aid of the other steps. There is no question any longer that, according to a wide variety of medical associations such as the American Association of Clinical Endocrinologists, According to Laurie Barclay, M.D., as published in the New AACE Guidelines for Prediabetes Management-Medscape 7/25/08 "As individual and as a society, we need to address those forces which are creating the epidemic of obesity, diabetes, and prediabetes." We all face the responsibility of spreading the word about this subject and encouraging our families—especially our children—to adopt a healthy diet to prevent diabetes.

your kids vitamins, and just about every child gets a vitamin daily (often masquerading as a cartoon character), and you probably take one, too. Clinical vitamin deficiency is rarely encountered in the United States today. In fact it's amazing that we don't have more vitamin insufficiency because our overall diet is poor in many respects—too many carbs and saturated fats. Still our diet does have enough nutrient value to prevent diseases, such as scurvy and beriberi, that were once common.

Vitamins are only one aspect or ingredient of nutraceuticals. Generally they are a blend of nutritious extracts of foods, vitamins, vegetables, minerals, herbs, amino acids, and other natural sources combined into a capsule, pill, or powder and used to make a shake or drink. Most of these products supplement medication, and they should not be depended on solely for treatment of diabetes. Most people who use these supplements believe they have some influence over chronic disease and that they provide a real benefit.

Understanding the Goals of Nutraceutical Therapy

There is a general agreement that vitamins and supplements help protect you and strengthen your system against diabetes, cardiovascular disease, and even cancer. Nutraceuticals have been clearly shown to help control lipid levels, blood pressure, and inflammation; raise body heat and increase metabolism; supplement antioxidants; provide thin and thick blood vessel wall protection; and aid with stress reduction and management of heart disease. Many medical specialists and wellness centers make them available to their patients. When you meet with a nutritionist, as described earlier, as part of your overall treatment, you should discuss which nutraceuticals should help you specifically, based on your stage of diabetes. Although many nutritionists and physicians don't promote natural therapies, you can explore this subject on your own if necessary or contact a physician who has experience in using supplements such as those discussed below. Most nutraceuticals are targeted, as you will see in the following.

Nutraceuticals Assist in Weight Loss
- Reduce hunger and appetite
- Increase metabolism and fat burning
- Control glucose and insulin levels
- Stop bingeing and craving

- Increase energy
- Reduce inflammation
- Improve gastrointestinal function

Nutraceuticals Reduce Cardiovascular and Diabetic Complications
- Hypertension
- Hyperlipidemia (high cholesterol, high blood triglycerides)
- Elevated homocysteine
- Increased blood coagulation or clot formation
- Oxidative stress
- Neuropathy
- Visual impairment
- Peripheral vascular disease
- Inflammation

Considering Nutraceuticals as a Valid Medical Treatment

Modern day clinical nutrition therapy has been confirmed by many scientific studies. They have reported its effectiveness in the management of multiple health problems. This aspect of medicine has evolved and is properly called nutri-pharmacology. I've reported on the use of nutrients as treatment for disease, for example, the use of niacin for hyperlipidemia. It's been described and confirmed as a nutrient to be used as a drug, hence the descriptive term "nutraceutical."

This part of Step Three can also be called cardio-nutrition and fits into lifestyle changes including diet, exercise, and stress reduction measures along with the nutraceuticals described below for the management of heart- and cardiovascular-related problems such as high blood pressure, high cholesterol, diabetes, weight management, fatigue, heart rhythm irregularities, congestive heart failure, and peripheral vascular disease.

Mainstream medicine has now embraced lifestyle changes to improve health, but many doctors are reluctant to prescribe supplements beyond folic acid and omega-3 fatty acids. Both the American Heart Association and American Diabetes Association have advised diets high in omega-3 fatty acids. Diets high in fiber have been also recommended by the American Society of Hypertension. They have not advised taking fiber supplements.

Adding nutraceuticals to your medication regimen is neither alternative medication nor holistic; it is actually integrative medicine, which is widely practiced by most physicians today. In integrative medicine, doctors try to work closely with patients, pursuing a number of treatments. A broken leg, for example, would be treated with a cast, perhaps surgery, and some time on crutches. However some doctors will also suggest taking certain supplements or vitamins that are thought to speed healing or increase bone strength. This combination of proven, science-backed medical treatment and the use of nontraditional medicine for prevention and enhancement is being accepted as government-sponsored studies are released. In fact, the U.S. National Institutes of Health has its own division—the National Center for Complimentary and Alternative Medicine—to study and issue scientific and advisory reports on these supplements and programs such as Ayurvedic medicine, a form of holistic medicine that is widely practiced in India.

Today, most well-informed people want the option of natural therapies. With regards to diabetes and especially weight loss, there are many well-researched options. The supplement program is an integral part of the unique diabetic weight management system used in my practice.

Recommended Vitamins or Supplements

I recommend the following nutraceuticals as part of a sound food and nutrition program.

In general, nutraceuticals are not prescribed by brand name, but by category. Because they are over-the-counter medications, shop around for the best price. These supplements are widely available at a discount in some superstores or can be found on the Internet. Dosages may vary, and generally the dosage should be as recommended by the manufacturer.

Magnesium: Magnesium is a critical mineral for people with diabetes and for everyone. Magnesium is involved in more than 300 enzymatic reactions in the body. From a cardiovascular point of view, magnesium is critical because it modulates blood pressure, heart rhythm, and heart performance. It is a key agent in enhancing the ability of the heart muscle fibers to contract, helping to stop arrhythmias, and helping to control blood pressure naturally.

In addition, magnesium is a part of glucose and insulin reactions, and that is why it is so important for people with diabetes. Magnesium has been found to be lower in people with fatigue, and it is a significant element in your body's management of bone metabolism.

Magnesium is especially important in people with diabetes since they have cardiovascular problems, and magnesium has also been shown to have anti-inflammatory benefits. Magnesium is also selectively excreted by diabetics from renal impairment, and this is significant because magnesium is important not only for glucose and insulin but for cardiovascular function.

Magnesium is often taken with calcium, but you can also buy it separately in the form of magnesium chelates, oxide, citrate, taurate, glycinate, and other preparations. Some people, like myself, prefer to use magnesium orotate because it works quickly in the body. Magnesium citrate is useful for people who suffer from constipation because it enhances bowel function.

Omega-3 fatty acids: Omega-3 supplements are of great significance to people with and without diabetes alike. Diets high in omega-3 have been recommended by the American Heart Association and the American Diabetes Association. Nowadays, with the lack of omega-3 content in many types of farmed fish, the toxicity in fish with PCBs (polychlorinated biphenyl), and the high level of mercury in certain deepwater fish, it is absolutely essential to take a high potency omega-3 supplement. At least 1,000 to 3,000 milligrams of the EPA portion of an omega-3 supplement are critical for most individuals for cardiovascular protection, and higher requirements are necessary for its potent triglyceride-lowering effect.

Cardiac benefits of omega-3 supplementation include reducing triglycerides and inflammation, stabilizing heart rhythm, reducing the incidence of sudden cardiac death, and reducing blood clots. This is especially important for people with diabetes since their lipid profile makes them more prone to accelerate arteriosclerosis and thrombosis.

Additional benefits of omega-3 supplementation include its enhancement of brain function, including improvement of memory and mood, and reduction in the progression of macular degeneration, dementia, and possibly even Alzheimer's disease.

Recently the American Association of Endocrinologists indicated that omega-3 supplements also enhance fat oxidation, and this makes them an important addition to the diabetic weight loss program. People who are over-weight as well as diabetic have a high incidence of arthritis and joint problems, for which high dose omega-3 supplementation is of great benefit. Omega-3 supplementation will also improve irritable bowel and inflammatory bowel disease.

Chromium: Chromium is one of the most commonly used and widely researched supplements in the area of glucose metabolism and diabetes. Studies have revealed that the majority of people measured for chromium content in the blood are deficient, and the average American's diet is low in chromium. This is a particularly serious problem for people with prediabetes and diabetes, since chromium is important in metabolism for glucose and insulin control.

Chromium allows glucose transport into the cells, and without it insulin is not effectively used. Studies have shown many metabolic benefits of chromium beyond glucose control, including improvement in body composition and lipid levels. There has been no real documentation that it assists with weight loss.

I recommend taking chromium GTF, with the chromium in the nicotinate form, and combined with vanadium.

Vanadium: This is another mineral important for glucose and insulin action. Experts believe that vanadium mimics the action of insulin in the body, and the key action of insulin is in glucose transport into muscles and fat cells. Studies have revealed that vanadium stimulates glucose uptake in cells, and it appears to be effective when there is insulin resistance and, therefore, reduces insulin resistance. Chromium and vanadium are extremely important in glucose and insulin metabolism, along with magnesium, zinc, and the B vitamin biotin.

Phaseolamin (phaseolus vulgaris): For someone with diabetes who has trouble controlling blood glucose and also reducing carbohydrate intake, phaseolamin is a natural carbohydrate blocker. This extract of the white kidney bean has been well researched. It slows down the digestion of starch by inhibiting alpha-amylase, which is an enzyme that breaks down starch so it can be more fully absorbed by the body. This carbohydrate blocking thus reduces the glycemic index of foods, reduces the number of carbohydrates that are actually ingested, and overall has been shown to help with blood glucose control and weight loss.

Fiber: It is impossible for most of us to take in large amounts of fiber in the diet. Fiber supplementation with products such as psyllium, oat pectin, fiber glucans, or apple pectin has been successfully used in a number of weight loss programs. Fiber supplements of any type have been shown to be very effective in reducing the glycemic effect of food (controlling your blood sugar), lowering cholesterol and therefore lowering glucose levels, detoxifying and helping with weight loss, which are all fantastic advantages for someone on a diabetic weight management system. Beta-glucans from oat have also been documented to help lower LDL cholesterol.

Digestive enzymes and probiotics: One of the significant roadblocks to weight loss is digestive problems. It is not unusual for overweight people with diabetes who are on a poor diet high in sugars and calories, who smoke and/ or drink alcohol, or are using drugs to have gastrointestinal problems, including indigestion, bloating, heartburn, acid reflux, and GERD. Additionally, because of toxic diet and frequent use of antibiotics and other medications, there is often an overgrowth of the yeast *Candida* in the intestines, often leading to fatigue, gas, and bloating.

For people with problems like these, I first recommend digestive enzymes to aid in the digestion of starches, proteins, and fats, frequently underproduced by the pancreatic stress. I also recommend probiotics, including good acidophilus formulas such as the Ohira and Shahani types. I've used these in my practice with tremendous benefit in helping people relieve gastrointestinal problems and therefore improving their ability to successfully enter a weight loss program.

Vitamin D: I recommend vitamin D for all of my patients, especially the 25-hydroxy vitamin D known as vitamin D_3, which is the bioactive form of vitamin D. Vitamin D has been prominent in the news lately. A study reported by the National Public Health Institute in Helsinki, Finland, found that men with the highest vitamin D levels in their blood were least likely to have developed type 2 diabetes twenty-two years later. Recent reports also indicate that vitamin D reduces insulin resistance.

The benefits of vitamin D go well beyond its benefit in bone biochemistry. Recent studies have shown that lower levels of vitamin D are associated with a higher risk of heart attack and decreased life span. These studies have also revealed that vitamin D has an anti-inflammatory and immuno-enhancing effect. It has been effective in preventing many types of cancer, and it's also important for prevention of autoimmune problems. An adequate intake of vitamin D is critical for everyone, especially people with diabetes, since low levels of vitamin D should probably now be considered an additional coronary risk factor.

Resveratrol: This nutritional supplement has been very prominent in the news for a number of reasons. This supplement first hit the headlines in stories about the French paradox. Studies have shown the French to enjoy a reduced cardio-vascular (heart attack) risk, in spite of some not-so-healthy lifestyle habits such as high fat intake and cigarette smoking. This is felt to be partly due to the antioxidants in the red wine they consume, of which resveratrol is a major component. The bioactive compounds in resveratrol seem to be very anti-inflammatory, with potent antioxidant benefits. They also prevent the platelets in the blood from sticking together and causing clotting problems.

Resveratrol was on the front page in a 2007 *New York Times* story. Harvard researchers reported that mice who were given a high fat, high calorie diet developed heart disease, diabetes, and liver damage. However, when they were supplemented with resveratrol, none of these problems occurred. The animals became leaner and had no evidence of blood sugar alterations or liver problems. Resveratrol is now being reported in the diabetic literature as something that could possibly be an additional help, since it seems to reduce insulin resistance and help with weight loss. It is also very effective as a brain-protecting nutrient, and it's considered to be a longevity nutrient. Its cardiovascular, neurologic, and diabetic potential benefits are why I use it to treat all of the patients coming into my centers.

Coenzyme Q10: Coenzyme Q10 (CoQ10) is a critical micronutrient to be considered in a diabetes management program. It does not specifically help with weight loss, other than the fact that it has an energy enhancing capability.

Coenzyme Q10 is not a vitamin since it is produced in scarce amounts in the body. A multitude of studies have shown the cardiovascular benefits of coenzyme Q10 or ubiquinone. This nutrient is very important for mitochondrial function, because it enhances ATP production in the mitochondria, which is the energy-producing portion of the cell. This is critical since the heart works 24/7. Studies have shown that people with reduced heart function, cardiomyopathy, and left ventricular dysfunction have reduced levels of coenzyme Q10, and there is improvement in heart function with supplementation.

Q10 is also a potent antioxidant against LDL cholesterol, which is one of the critical initiating factors of progressive arteriosclerosis. Q10 has been shown to be helpful in blood pressure regulation through its insulin-modulating effects, and it is critical for people who have reduced energy and fatigue. I always recommend Q10 for my patients with diabetes, especially those with heart problems and fatigue. Studies have also shown that it is important for neurocognitive function and prevention of periodontal disease. It has been reported to help with migraines, too, and overall it's one of my key cardiovascular enhancing nutrients.

Aged garlic (Kyolic): This special form of garlic does not necessarily aid weight loss, but it enhances multiple systems that are critical for the people with diabetes. There are thousands of scientific research reports on aged garlic. It's very important for cardiovascular function since it acts as a vascular relaxant, decreasing adrenaline and dilating the blood vessels. This helps with blood pressure. It also has been shown to help lower cholesterol, improve the lining of the blood vessels, and improve glucose regulation. It reduces cortisol and reduces oxidative stress. Increased cortisol leads to nerve and kidney damage. Studies on aged garlic reported at the experimental biology meeting in 2008 found that the extract actually slowed down the progression of arteriosclerosis and enhanced blood flow.

D-Ribose: D-Ribose is a five-carbon sugar that has been researched and is used extensively by cardiovascular nutritionists. It's one of my key cardio-vascular nutrients—along with omega-3 fatty acids, magnesium, coenzyme Q10, and aged garlic. D-Ribose is a nutrient that has been shown to be very effective in the areas of fatigue and cardiac function. Studies have shown that people with impaired left ventricular function, congestive heart failure, and cardiomyopathy are markedly improved by D-Ribose supplementation. This simple sugar, which does not affect blood sugar (in fact it lowers blood sugar since it acts differently than glucose), has been shown to enhance ATP production in the mitochondria, the cellular powerhouse. Additional studies of chronic fatigue have indicated that supplementation with D-Ribose markedly reduces fatigue, muscle aches, and fibromyalgia. It is this function of enhancing energy that makes D-Ribose so important for people with diabetes, since diabetes is what I call an "energy crisis disease."

The nutrient does not specifically help with weight loss, but by enhancing energy it allows you to become more active, start to exercise, and have your body and cells function in a much more normal and improved fashion.

Vitamin K$_2$: A thirty-six-month study released in late 2008 indicated that vitamin K supplementation (usually in the form of food high in the vitamin) "may reduce the progression of insulin resistance in older men," according to the November 2008 issue of *Diabetes Care*. It did not have as dramatic an effect in women.

Vitamin K has also shown to have potentially remarkable capacity for reducing risk of atherosclerosis.

There are two forms of vitamin K: K_1 and K_2. The difference is their chemical structure. K_1 usually is found in green leafy vegetable such as spinach, lettuce, and parsley. K_2 is found in fermented products such as cheeses and also in butter and eggs. Depending on their relative absorption time in the body they can be labeled MK4 and MK7. (I advise the use of K_2 [menquone-7] for every patient at my centers.)

Vitamin K also seems to help promote blood coagulation (clotting), so if you take blood thinners, it's especially important to discuss it with your doctor first.

Other Supplements and Nutraceuticals to Consider

You may wish to read up on and research the following supplements and discuss them with your doctor and nutritionist.

Nutraceuticals for Glucose, Insulin, Diabetes, and Weight Management
The products in capitals are the ones often used and recommended by the author.

- MAGNESIUM
- CHROMIUM/VANADIUM
- OMEGA-3 FATTY ACIDS
- PHASEOLUS VULGARIS (WHITE BEAN EXTRACT)
- FIBER SUPPLEMENTS/OAT BETA-GLUCAN
- DIGESTIVE ENZYMES/PROBIOTICS
- VITAMIN D
- RESVERATROL
- B vitamins
- DHEA
- Banana leaf extract
- Garcinai cambogia
- Gymnema sylvestre

Reminder: Do not take any of these supplements without discussing them with your physician because there can be possible interactions with your medications. The same is true of traditional medications.

- Bitter melon
- Zinc
- Biotin
- Selenium
- Cinnamon
- Ginseng
- Lipoic acid
- Green tea extract
- Fenugreek
- Glucomannan
- Hoodia gordoni
- Citrus aurantium
- Coleus forskohlii
- Asian pumpkin extract

Nutraceuticals for Cardiovascular Problems, Lipis, Hypertension, Inflammation, Thrombosis, and Homocysteine

The products in capitals are the ones often used and recommended by the author.

- OMEGA-3 FATTY ACIDS
- FIBER SUPPLEMENTS
- COENZYME Q10
- MAGNESIUM/POTASSIUM
- VITAMIN D
- Potassium
- Taurine
- Arginine
- Hawthorne
- Antioxidant vitamins
- B vitamins
- Red yeast rice/policosanol (This one is controversial.)
- Plant phytosterols, guggul
- Niacin
- Nattokinase
- Plant phytonutrients
- Pomegranate

- Vitamin E/tocotrienols
- Flavanoids
- Turmeric
- Green tea extract
- DHA/Gingko
- Phosphatdyl serine
- Orosine

LOOK BEYOND THE NUTRACEUTICALS

Lately, attention has been drawn to hormonal factors in diabetes and obesity (sometimes called diabesity) that have to be aggressively treated with nondiabetic medications or nutraceuticals. Frequently, people with diabetes have hypothyroidism or early-stage hypothyroidism (insufficient thyroid hormone). Recent publications have indicated that a higher range of thyroid stimulating hormone, even a level within normal range, can be associated with the inability to lose weight.

Frequently seen with hypothyroidism is adrenal fatigue and adrenal hormone depression, for which DHEA replacement therapy can be effective in increasing energy and reducing visceral adiposity.

Many men with prediabetes and diabetes have testosterone deficiency. This is a concern that must be managed in diabetic men. Administration of the testosterone hormone helps the insulin resistance of diabetes, and it also improves endurance, depression, energy levels, and libido, and it lessens erectile dysfunction.

Other problems that are often addressed in people with diabetes are brain fog and intestinal dysbiosis, which are by-products of high glucose levels. For this, certain diets that reduce allergens such as wheat or gluten are quite effective in reducing weight as well. In addition, yeast infections such as *Candida albicans* are often found in people with diabetes and must be treated.

KEEP MOVING FOR WEIGHT LOSS

To this point we've discussed how you can defeat the natural roadblocks that challenge you as a diabetic with education, targeted medications, and a diet that balances protein, limited carbohydrates, and other healthy foods. Now we will concentrate on the fact that exercise plays as important a role as the other parts of the Five-Step Plan as a control mechanism for prediabetes or type 2 diabetes. Exercise can literally blast through roadblocks.

The good news is that according to many studies published by organizations such as the American Diabetes Association and the American Council on Exercise, the latest research has put exercise at the forefront in the prevention, control, and treatment of diabetes because it decreases insulin resistance. Following regular exercise training, cells can better respond to insulin and appropriately take up glucose out of the blood.

Virtually every study also indicates that exercise is specifically advantageous for people with type 2 diabetes over the long run and attacks visceral fat and your lipid levels.

In addition, the studies show that diet and exercise together are even more effective than dieting alone. And dieting without exercising—especially in the elderly—causes people to lose valuable muscle mass.

The most important thing to understand is that there is definitive proof that if you have prediabetes, exercise can keep you from developing diabetes—even if all you do is some very moderate form of exercise on a regular basis. Other studies have indicated that even limited periods of exercise (e.g., two months) will have a positive effect on your A1C value, and it can be significant. In one study, A1C levels dropped from 8.31 to 7.65, despite the fact that there was no appreciable weight loss in the two groups of participants in the study.

While your exercise program does not have to be ambitious, it does require a commitment. Every prediabetic or diabetic, and possibly concomitant cardiovascular disease, must exercise. Exercising for the rest of your life is a critical cornerstone of the wall you are building to protect yourself from further damage to your health and blood glucose levels. Though exercise is usually an adjunct to taking medications, your exercise program might lead to reduced medication levels.

UNDERSTAND THE BENEFITS OF EXERCISE

There is absolutely no question, given the studies reported above, that regular, even moderate to medium-level, exercise has a significant effect on diabetic management and can delay or prevent prediabetes from becoming type 2 diabetes. Dozens of studies indicate that as rates of diabetes mellitus and obesity continue to increase, physical activity continues to be a fundamental form of therapy. Exercise influences several aspects of diabetes, including blood glucose concentrations, insulin action, and cardiovascular risk factors.

Exercise, except in people who have injuries or severe health problems such as advanced heart disease, pulmonary conditions, or orthopedic restrictions, is always beneficial, no matter what level you can manage. Here are the benefits of at least 30 minutes of exercise a day, 3 to 5 days a week, to people with diabetes:

- Reduced blood sugar levels—especially in people with type 2 diabetes
- Halted transformation from prediabetes to type 2 diabetes or even to insulin dependence
- Reduced adipose fat levels
- Lowered insulin resistance, enabling your cells to respond to insulin

- Controlled (and improved) cholesterol, triglycerides, and other lipid levels
- Stress relief (very important!)
- Attaining proper weight/BMI for your frame
- Stronger immunity from disease
- Lowered blood pressure
- Reduced brain fog and increased alertness
- Slowed aging (Studies are beginning to appear that indicate that exercise may be able to affect your genetic structure, reversing aging. While these are only small studies, they are significant, and they suggest that exercise might be a secret weapon for the life extension/antiaging movement.)
- Improved mental health

But why does exercise help? One of the unique features of diabetes is that regaining your health is largely up to you. You have to monitor your glucose levels, and maintain a diet that balances your nutritional needs. Now you've been told that you have to add exercise, and despite the clear benefits explained above, exercise is often on the bottom of the list of things you'd like to do. However, as you come to understand why exercise works, how it affects you biologically, this will help you overcome inertia and procrastination and maybe even make you eager to step on the treadmill or get out your walking shoes.

You already know that when you eat certain foods, insulin is released and transported to your muscles and other organs to stimulate activity. Exercise does the same thing, but through a different process that also helps you lose weight. In other words, there are two ways that you can get glucose into your bloodstream and to its target: proper diet is one and exercise is the other.

Studies now show that any period of exercise will raise the intake of glucose to various key muscle groups, cells, and adipose tissue. This is accomplished through a glucose transporter, known as GLUT4, moving glucose through your bloodstream. This is a self-regulating system that responds to your workout—a good walk or other sustained activity. Lowering glucose levels builds muscle and increases insulin sensitivity through more effective muscular function.

Keep in mind that you are exercising for a couple reasons: to control your glucose levels and to reduce your risk of death from cardiovascular disease. Exercise will keep your cardiovascular system working properly to reduce your blood pressure, lower cholesterol levels, and most important, help you reduce your weight. All of this will come with even a moderate exercise program.

GET MOVING

Adding exercise to your life for anyone who has diabetes, is overweight, or has any other cardiovascular problem is seemingly a no-brainer, especially given the overwhelming scientific evidence of the benefits. But how to start, what to do, and how to make it a true part of your life may be mini-roadblocks. Don't despair: Exercise options are everywhere.

Exercise for diabetes control does not require expensive equipment and can be as simple as you wish. Your exercise goals should be simple: Make effective exercise a built-in part of your daily life because it always has benefit no matter the level.

The general rule is to begin slowly and build; this is not a sudden onslaught. You might have some natural anxiety about exercise and whatever you choose to do should not overwhelm you because adjusting diet and medications alone can be big enough stressors.

Checking with Your Doctor First

Let me re-emphasize how important it is for your doctor to review any sort of exercise program. When you talk to an exercise instructor and your medical professional, they should first do a complete physical assessment to ensure that you can safely begin any type of workout. If like many people with diabetes, you also have cardiovascular problems or they are suspected, you should consider the following:

- If you are entering a combined, supervised program for diabetes and heart trouble, the coordinator or nurse should take a complete history, going over your current medications and concomitant illness.
- Get clearance from a cardiologist before beginning to exercise. In acute situations such as after a heart attack or angioplasty, a cardio monitored program is advised.
- In general you should begin with light exercise, perhaps 5 to 10 minutes a day, and start on a diet that enables you to establish new eating patterns.

If you join a program, the main goal should be to teach you how to exercise properly and to establish some baselines. For example, you want to establish a target heart rate in a supervised exercise environment so that you will be able to work out on your own. You may be asked to wear a telemetry monitor, and your blood pressure will be taken at intervals while you walk on a treadmill. Of course, if you have diabetes, you should monitor your glucose levels before and after you exercise, depending on your diabetic status, to avoid any sudden sugar level drops.

Exercising with Caution

Despite the obvious benefits to glucose control through exercise, you can't simply jump onto the treadmill, lie down on the weight bench, or start mega-walks circling the park numerous times. Too much exercise—especially as you start—can have two negative effects, which ironically are the exact opposite of each other: hyperglycemia or hypoglycemia.

Hypoglycemia occurs if your blood sugar suddenly drops and leaves you feeling hungry, dizzy, weak, anxious, lightheaded, and even confused. Generally, only people with diabetes become hypoglycemic, but it can be a side effect of medication or symptom of some other underlying medical problem. One way to prevent this is to learn the proper foods to eat before exercise: a combination of protein with some carbs.

Hyperglycemia is the exact opposite and signifies that your blood sugar has risen beyond normal and is extremely high. If your blood sugar levels shoot up, you will feel thirsty (and perhaps hungry), urinate frequently, possibly experience "dry-mouth," and
in extreme cases feel sleepy and unable to focus.

What sort of exercise causes either of these dangerous conditions? It's hard to predict because the conditions that might cause one can also provoke the other, and the chemistry of these reactions is not fully understood. So stay aware of your blood sugar levels when you begin exercising. Almost always there will be a drop in glucose levels after exercise.

It is generally not necessary to check your blood glucose unless you are having symptoms. If your blood glucose becomes too low, you can have a small amount of carbohydrates with protein or a glucose tablet. If it goes too high, management depends on your specific drug therapy.

Always let your physician know that you intend to begin any sort of exercise program that he or she has not already approved.

These effects should not be a reason to avoid exercise because, as stated above, there is definitive evidence that exercise is a key factor in reducing type 2 diabetes effects. To give yourself a safety margin, you can wear a Medic Alert bracelet that indicates you are diabetic, exercise with a partner, and make sure that you see your doctor before you initiate any type of exercise program.

Unsafe exercising can be as dangerous as not exercising at all. Keep the following few things in mind to keep from hurting yourself or overdoing it:

- Warm up before you begin: Stretch and move your arms around to loosen your muscles and improve your range of motion, and begin slowly.
- Wear loose clothing to allow you to perspire, letting your skin breathe and keeping your temperature lower.
- Keep the FITT formula (see page 121) in mind, noting the frequency, intensity, and duration each time you exercise so that you don't do too much.

don't forget your feet

Good shoes are important in almost any form of exercise, and even more so for people with diabetes. Here are a few tips from sports medicine expert Elizabeth Quinn on picking good exercise shoes:

- Consult a doctor or podiatrist first if necessary, and if you wear an orthotic, bring it along.
- Know your foot type (flat, wide, pointing in or out?) and choose shoes that offer appropriate support.
- Look for shoes with cushioning for shock absorption.
- Make sure shoes bend at the ball of the foot.
- Shop in the afternoon, when the feet are slightly swollen.
- Wear your sport socks when trying on shoes.
- Always try on both shoes and lace them as you would for activity.
- Make sure the heel is snug and does not slide.
- Check that you have a thumb's width between your longest toe and the tip of the toe box.
- Walk (or jog) around the store.
- Buy shoes that feel good immediately; you should never have to break in a pair of athletic shoes.
- If you have severe foot problems, consult your podiatrist.

If you are committed to your exercise program and begin to see the evidence described earlier, your blood sugars will come down and then the only excuses you will have are the ones you make up! You don't have to exercise every day to have an effect. You can limit your walking or any other activity to 20 to 30 minutes, 3 or 4 days a week, but try to make sure at least two of those sessions are back to back.

- Choose the type in relation to the problem you have, whether it's controlling your diabetes and hypertension or promoting your heart health. Talk to your doctor.
- Cool down as you finish your workout: For example, walk slower to get your heartbeat back to normal.

CHOOSE THE BEST EXERCISE FOR YOU

What kind of exercise works? The answer to this is really quite simple: anything that you can do that gets your heart pumping a bit faster than normal for a relatively short period of time.

Exercise has often been equated with athletic training, but no one expects you to turn into a marathon runner, although many heart patients have recovered to the point where they do participate in competitive sports, including running, softball, golf, and tennis.

You have so many exercise options today that it's hard to avoid falling over gyms, workout programs, "as-seen-on-TV" machines, classes, yoga institutes, and multimedia products. Before you invest in anything, mold the elements of the basics described in the following pages into a program that is likely to help you to succeed on your own, perhaps starting with exercise at your local park.

Walking: A Great Place to Begin

You've probably heard these ideas before, but if you actually do things like take the stairs more often and park far from the supermarket door or even walk the mall (avoiding the food court) for 30 to 40 minutes, you have started doing something very important. You've begun to make exercise in its most basic form—walking—a habit! Once you get hooked, you'll look forward to it and make it part of your everyday life.

"Right," you say, unconvinced. "What about bad weather?" You live in the north, and it rains or snows on and off for months. Walk in your office on your lunch, walk in the stairwells if you can and, again, the mall. Find out when the local high school or YMCA gym is available for walking. It's usually a small cost, if any.

There is no question that simple walking has enormous benefits, especially if you can't afford equipment or are not cleared for anything else. Studies carried out at Massachusetts General Hospital found that when women were given different aerobic exercise for several months, walking was, by far, their favorite. One good thing about walking is that it is a low-impact activity, and it is easy to get back into it when you've been a couch potato for a long time. Just stand up and take one step after another.

Walking has additional benefits. It's a low-impact exercise that increases bone mass and has a lasting effect on bone density, which is particularly important to women. A more high-impact exercise might stimulate more bone mass growth; however, walking is less painful than a high-impact workout. Walking before eating (especially before large holiday meals) can help protect your heart from the effect of fatty foods.

Exploring Other Exercise Options

When it comes to exercise, you have many more choices, as described below, and you might have attempted some of these in the past. Even so, with a new diet (Step Three) and proper medication (Step Two), these activities will work. As always, have your doctor evaluate what you can do and what you like to do and ask for safe recommendations. Here are some of those choices:

- Aerobic training—walking, swimming, treadmills
- Cross training—resistance and aerobic—walking, running, and using light weights.
- Serious weight training—working on one or two body parts per machine (Bear in mind that abdominal training alone will not help you get rid of visceral fat.)
- Circuit training
- Exercise classes
- Kickboxing
- Dance aerobics
- Yoga

be a tortoise, not a hare

You've heard the old saying: Slow and steady wins the race. Well, it may also burn more calories, at least in the long run. Researchers at Maastricht University in the Netherlands concluded that people who engage in moderate physical activity, such as walking and biking, had the highest overall physical activity levels. Their study of thirty men and women over a two-week period also revealed that those who exercised vigorously for short periods of time compensated for that activity by spending a greater part of their day being sedentary. Sure, vigorous exercise burns more calories, but the moderate exercisers tended to be more active overall.

Combining Aerobic and Resistance Exercise

An effective program should consist of a mixture of both aerobic and resistance exercising. You may have tried commercial, club-type programs before that included this dual approach, yet you slipped back to your old self after some initial success. Nothing is more discouraging than being promised a buffed body in three months, and ninety days later you still look the same in the mirror. But what you don't realize is that you might have achieved a real benefit to your diabetes. Weight loss takes time, but better blood sugars, on the other hand, can occur very quickly. And the proof will be in your "numbers."

Aerobic exercise is literally any activity that increases the rate and depth of your breathing, raises your heart rate, and uses your large muscle groups. The most frequent forms of aerobic exercise are walking, running, biking, and swimming. To be beneficial, a regular program of exercise begins in small increments and builds up to 30 minutes a day, 3 to 5 days per week. To ensure safety, any man older than age forty with diabetes and heart disease and any woman older than age fifty should have their exercise program reviewed by their cardiologist.

Resistance training is the opposite of aerobic training. The idea is to strengthen and tone your body or parts of your body. In general, light-weight training or use of machines that impose resistance on your arms or legs are used. Elastic bands and the Nautilus machines are popular.

The only difference for a diabetic is that it is an essential part of diabetic management to improve insulin sensitivity.

Aim for at least 20 minutes of resistance exercises 3 times per week.

Exercising with Type 2 Diabetes

According to the American Council on Exercise, if you have type 2 diabetes, you should follow the following exercise guidelines, which are the same ones used for prevention of cardiac problems:

- Cardiovascular exercise: Aim for 30 minutes of moderate-intensity exercise (walking and other non-weight-bearing activities such as water aerobics and cycling are good choices) 3 to 5 days per week. Daily exercise, however, is highly recommended.
- Resistance training: You can use a dumbbell program with 2 to 10-pound (900 g to 4.5 kg) barbells at home, following instructions from exercise books or the store where you purchase them. For more advanced weight training, work with a professional trainer on specific body parts, including chest, back, biceps, triceps, shoulders, abdominals, hamstrings, calves, and quadriceps.
- Circuit training for resistance in a gym
- Rowing machine
- Elliptical machines
- Flexibility exercises: At least two or three days per week, stretch major muscle groups to the point of tightness (not pain) for 15 to 30 seconds, 2 to 4 times per stretch. Also, most fitness experts suggest some sort of stretching routine prior to any workout.

You may also need a specific exercise program designed for your unique needs. For example, there is a program for women who suffer from leg problems such as cramping caused by peripheral artery disease. Your doctor can point you in the right direction if this is the case.

Controlling Exercise Intensity

Part of any exercise program is ensuring that it actually provides benefit. Your exercise program must have three basic components, according to Michael Crawford, MS, the supervisor of cardio-rehabilitation programs at the Cleveland Clinic. "You have to have aerobic exercise, and it must be regular, and, it must be above all safe."

The FITT program is a well-known approach for keeping track of your exercise efforts and includes:

F = Frequency

I = Intensity

T = Type of exercise

T = Time or duration

The FITT program is often worked into a recovery program. In the case of my coauthor, Lawrence Chilnick, he used it after open heart surgery. (He is also a diabetic who needed to lose weight.) During recovery from heart surgery it's important to go through both a supervised, formal cardo-rehab program and a personal, at home exercise program. While the cardio-recovery center had its own customized program, at home it was harder for him to keep to a program. He was, however given some good advice, "Try to do every exercise at home more each day." Using the FITT concept, he kept a daily record of his at-home exercise and could clearly see his progress.

Another way to track exercise intensity is with a widely used device called the Rated-Perceived Exertion (RPE) Scale. This scale is a simple way to measure the intensity of your activity or exercise. While the scale runs from 0 to 10 in benefit (10 being the most intense), it is somewhat subjective and uses phrases matched to numbers to help you measure your workout. Here's how it works.

The Rated Perceived Exertion Scale (RPE)

How hard is your activity?

1	Not at all	6	Heavy
1.5	Just noticeable	7	
2	Very light	8	Very heavy
3	Light	9	
4	Moderate	10	Very, very heavy (maximum)
5	Somewhat heavy		

In general, keep your exercise level between 3 and 4, although you must first clear the type and intensity of exercise with your doctor. With this scale, you can keep track of how exercise is affecting you. If you find after a month or two that your exercise intensity is now a 2 instead of a 3, you can work out more often or a little more intensely. One expert says that an ideal level of workout would mean that "you are able to talk, but not sing while doing it."

Integrating Exercise into Your Life

No matter what method or equipment you use, I suggest following a few guidelines. (1) Involve your kids and your spouse or partner in working physical activity into your daily life. Exercise for heart health does not require anything more than an activity that gets your RPE up to 3 to 4, 5 or 6 times per week. The level you need to get to is up to you and your doctor, but 30 minutes a day, 3 to 5 times per week is a minimum. (2) Walk to the store and walk up stairs whenever you can. (3) Clean the house, work in the yard; it doesn't matter. You've been much less active than you should be, and that's affected your heart. You will be surprised how quickly you begin to recover.

Crawford suggests that you should spend a minimum of 30 minutes in each exercise session and aim for 3 to 5 days a week. You can go beyond that under careful supervision. This will help a great deal in weight loss. Remember that exercise alone will not help you lose weight. If you can put together a longer exercise regimen with a diet of reduced calories, that's the best thing you can do for yourself as a diabetic.

The ultimate goal is to expend a minimum of 1,000 calories per week with physical activity for health benefits, or 2,000 calories per week for weight loss. Keep in mind that these are goals that you should work up to gradually over time.

What about those exercise machines? You might already have an expensive piece of exercise equipment sitting in the family room or bedroom, mainly serving as a clothing rack or dust collector. It's also likely to be a stationary bike, since that has traditionally been the most popular piece of exercise equipment. However, exercise equipment has changed to meet the needs of its market, and much of that market is people who need to rescue themselves from diabetes and lose weight. This new equipment industry is also aimed at those looking for stress reduction, body toning, and overall fitness.

To meet your needs as a person with diabetes and/or heart disease, there are new versions of treadmills and exercycles, and new devices such as the elliptical exercise machine, that can provide a solid aerobic workout.

There are some very good reasons to invest in a piece of exercise equip-ment, even if your old stationary bike experience was not a good one. Today's exercise equipment is programmable to help you maximize its aerobic effect. In addition, much of it is reasonably priced for the ever-expanding, longer-living, fitness-oriented population.

Having the right mini-gym in your home may help you develop and maintain the habit of exercising. It may become a magnet for you and a great opportunity to involve your family in your weight loss program. Letting older children use the equipment encourages them to form a routine that that will benefit them throughout their lives.

Purchasing Exercise Equipment

The place to begin when making a decision on an equipment purchase is by asking your nutritional or cardio rehab supervisor and doctor for a recommendation. Another good source of information is a physical therapist who may be familiar with the newest versions and best brands of equipment. Other sources include Consumer Reports (www.consumerreports.org) and trade organizations such as the American Council on Fitness (www.acefitness.org). Also, search for websites that provide customer reviews.

My coauthor, Lawrence Chilnick, has had a very positive experience with equipment. At first, a treadmill was going to be an adjunct to the gym, but, instead, became a regular source of exercise. Recently, he added a recumbent exercise bike (see page 134) to break up routines and because it was easier on aging knees (also better for people with back problems). His total investment for both was under $1,000. Amortized over five years, it cost no more per year than the cost of joining a gym.

Treadmills

Treadmills are an excellent way to burn calories, get your leg muscles in shape, and keep track of how well you are doing. More than 11 million Americans use one regularly. Treadmills are, by far, the most popular pieces of exercise equipment and they provide the type of aerobic exercise you need.

Most treadmills give you a readout or graph of your distance, speed, calories burned, pulse, and other information. By increasing the incline of the treadmill surface, you can burn more calories. According to a study at the University of Wisconsin Medical School, a sixty-minute workout will burn up to 865 calories.

When you use a treadmill, you can increase either distance or speed, which enables you to slowly build up your tolerance. As you get healthier, you'll want to increase the speed because that will burn more calories. Or begin at one speed and raise it for a specific distance. Or slow down the speed for a half minute, and then increase your speed again—to a point past where you had been—for the same length of time. You can repeat this process for at least thirty minutes. By the time you finish, you'll know you've burned some calories.

Another reason you might like the treadmill is that you can exercise regardless of the weather, so you have no excuses. Some people like to read or watch TV while on the treadmill, but this is also a good opportunity to listen to music or audio books, which will help the time on the "track" pass more quickly.

Most important, the treadmill is a relatively safe device. It has a safety stop key and side rails, and you don't have to worry about the hazards of running outside. Make sure you buy a machine that has a long enough surface for running if you are going to use it for jogging.

Because treadmills are relatively expensive ($600 to $3,500), you have to choose the right one. When you go to buy one, wear sneakers and try out more than one machine, each for more than a few minutes. If the store won't demo it, go elsewhere. Make sure it's comfortable for you to walk on and that you can reach the controls easily. Finally, treadmills are not small, so consider where you are going to put the machine before you buy it.

Recumbent Exercise Bike

The second most popular exercise device is the recumbent bike, which is a bicycle-like device that has a seat on a level with the pedals and a backrest that provides support while you are pedaling. Similar to the treadmill, this machine provides the sort of aerobic exercise you need for cardio recovery or just plain exercise. To use it, you sit on the bike, adjust the pedals, and either program it or manually set the resistance to a level that gives you a good workout. Almost all of these bikes also have pulse and speed measurement functions.

There are multiple benefits to this machine. First is the cost: A top-of-the-line machine can be found for $250 to $350 and purchased online for less. Similar to treadmills, recumbent bikes are safe, but they put less of a strain on your knees, and they are quieter. They can also serve as your primary exercise machine because they can be used indoors.

Elliptical Exerciser

Elliptical exercisers are designed to give you a multifaceted workout, simulating everything from climbing stairs to a sort of cross-country skiing workout. Ellipticals provide a good overall resistance-type exercise. In 2003, sales of these machines jumped by 65 percent to 3.3 million home users. The basic activity comes from standing on two shoe-sized pedals that move in elliptical patterns, or "flattened circles." You climb up and down while pushing and pulling on handlebars. It takes a little while to get used to it, but it is not as hard as it sounds. The elliptical is an excellent machine because it is low impact and easy on your joints, plus you use both your arms and legs at the same time. The elliptical gives both your upper and lower body workouts with weight-bearing exercise, which helps protect you from osteoporosis.

Unfortunately, ellipticals are expensive. The models that work well at the gym usually cost about $5,000. Home machines cost $1,000 to $2,000, but they are not as well made as gym-quality machines and are not rated as highly by users.

When choosing an elliptical, you have to make sure it has adjustable and wide pedals, that the handlebars are designed so that you can reach them easily, and that it has the programmability that you need.

Other Useful Devices

You can find other exercise devices, but you should begin your recovery with one of the "big three" machines discussed above, along with other aerobic exercise of your choice. There are dozens of different abdominal and chinning/ total gym devices. These use angled boards with pulley devices that you use to raise yourself along the board. While this is good strengthening exercise, it is not aerobic, and while you will ultimately be able to lift your own weight, there is no way to increase the weight you are lifting.

Inversion tables, arm-curl machines, and other devices are designed to give you those six-pack abdominals. Unless you are completely cleared by your doctor and you use these machines in a supervised manner to start, stay away.

Another popular tool is a rowing machine, which can give you a good workout on many levels. It is especially good for muscle toning. Fans claim that it is as close to swimming as non-impact exercises get. The downside of the rowing machine is that it can be hard on your back and can aggravate previous injuries.

exercise mats

I strongly recommend having some sort of mat under your treadmill or other equipment, and it's a good idea to ask that one be included in the sale.

Mats are also an obvious way to avoid getting hurt while doing exercises such as yoga or Pilates and are strongly recommended. There are literally dozens of types made of foam or cushioned tiles that will protect you from injury and your exercise space from damage. The main difference between the mats is price, and they usually cost between $35 and $60, depending on size and portability.

Beyond these, there are resistance bands, giant exercise balls, dumbbells, and traditional bicycles. Biking is great aerobic exercise, but if you are just recovering from heart surgery or a heart attack, you may be told to wait for a while before starting. There are dozens of good bikes for anyone of any age. I have met many people who ride bikes as part of their weight loss program; however, bike use is limited by the season or the weather. As good as a bike may be, it is not as effective as the devices mentioned above. And while it may be good for you when you are cleared to use one, a decent bike for comfort or fitness riding can cost between $300 and $600.

Joining a Health Club

Fitness clubs and community centers such as the YMCA are popular, but are they right for you? Many people apparently think so because there are 18,000 plus clubs in the United States and more than 32 million people shell out a considerable amount of money—$14.8 billion—each year to join. Not surprisingly, more than 50 percent of the members are women, and the largest segment of the over-55 group has joined to lose weight. A good source of information is the International Health Racquet & Sports Club Association at www.cms.ihrsa.org.

There is no question that health fitness clubs can be attractive, although some people are afraid of them since the club myth is that every member is buffed and built enough to smash through walls. This is simply not true. But relying on your own self-discipline alone can be daunting, and the "free trial" enticements from clubs and especially the branded programs can be compelling.

I've said some negative things about clubs and gyms because they don't have good records for long-term success. But there are people who like them. The clubs have also gotten the health/diet/diabetes weight loss/heart recovery message. More than half of clubs offer some sort of dedicated diet and nutrition counseling, along with heart-safe and health-related exercise programs. Another strategy clubs use is to align themselves with diet programs, such as Jenny Craig and Weight Watchers, that encourage exercise but have no formal exercise programs. They set up special low-impact exercise programs that don't involve weights, which is the usual attraction of a club.

The downside of clubs is that they tend to have high drop-out rates because people have to commit to go there for exercise and it interferes with last-minute business meetings, trips, or family responsibilities. If the club is your only exercise source, then it can quickly slip away.

Other considerations are cost and hours of operation. On the positive side, clubs can be a good place to meet people, and you can get good, professional instruction. They are good places for step and Pilates classes, which you might not do on your own. The decision to join a club is very much an individual one. If you feel comfortable with the idea of club membership and you can justify the cost of a club against investing in home equipment, then the choice is yours.

In the long run, you might want to invest in home equipment until you regain your heart health, then move to a club for a more intense workout.

CREATE YOUR OWN PROGRAM

Your exercise program does not have to be formidable and frightening. If you can find a friend or partner to exercise with, it might even be fun, and that will help you stick to it.

Here's an opening approach recommended by Crawford and other specialists that you can modify to fit your exercise needs:

Start with short-term goals. One positive about certain weight loss programs is that they are goal-oriented, and they use short-term motivators like weekly weigh-ins to mark progress. While this is not meant as an endorsement, this is one of the reasons programs like Weight Watchers have worked for some. It's very important to start with short-term goals when you begin exercise to measure your improvement. One reason that walking on the street or a treadmill is a good start in an exercise program is that with these exercises you can easily measure your progress.

It's important to remember to take your time, perhaps a few months, to develop your exercise habit. Don't expect results immediately. Ironically, some of the same physiologic, pleasure-seeking mechanisms that reinforce other bad habits kick in with exercise, but this is the best habit to have.

Choose the right time. Choose a good time to exercise, for you—not just when a club class begins—because you will, inevitably miss classes, and then you may possibly backslide and lose the benefit. We've all been there. It can't be said too many times: Make exercise a part of your daily routine. Make it a habit like brushing your teeth.

Mark your exercise as a daily appointment. Schedule exercise in your daily planner or PDA and keep to that schedule. If you miss one activity, do something else, such as taking a walk around the block, so that you continue to make exercise a habit and to ensure that the benefit and positive feelings you gain from it continue.

Keep a journal. In Step Three of the Five-Step Plan in this book, you are urged to keep track of what you eat. There is even more reason to keep an exercise log. This helps you keep track of how your RPE has changed and to see what type of exercise works for you best.

Have fun. While exercise and fun may seem to be mutually exclusive in your mind, they do not have to be. To begin with, you don't have to confine yourself to one form of exercise. Ride a bike one day, walk around the block three times the next day, and invite someone from your family or a buddy to play tennis the next. Rekindling an old skill, such as dancing or swimming, can break up the exercise pattern and motivate you even more.

YOUR NEW APPROACH TO LIFE LEADS TO WEIGHT LOSS

Change is never simple, but it does make a difference. For anyone who is at risk for type 2 diabetes or heart disease, making lifestyle changes is the final, critical step in the Five-Step Plan for diabetes control and weight loss. Lifestyle changes have been repeatedly proven to be one of the best ways to reduce the potential of prediabetes progressing to type 2 diabetes. Studies show that a better lifestyle can actually help you modify, reduce, and control the genetic roadblocks and risks you were born with.

Lifestyle change can also be the hardest part of weight loss for a prediabetic or type 2 diabetic. However, now that you are more aware of how diabetes affects you, making those changes will be easier and more likely to succeed.

Your own contribution to behavioral change may be the make-or-break factor. This doesn't mean you will be sent home from the doctor's office with an unbreakable list of do's and don'ts, rather a lifestyle plan you create together and that you implement, with a support system in place.

Your diabetes support system—especially where lifestyle change is concerned—should consist of a network of professionals in addition to your doctor, such as nutritionists or behavioral counselors, to help you with the natural feelings of depression or frustration that accompany lifestyle changes. It's vital that you also form a personal support team with family, friends, neighbors, or coworkers who can help you with dietary compliance and your medications. If this isn't possible, turn to a medical or dietary professional for help. In all almost all cases, lifestyle modification is difficult to start, but it's easier to put into effect once you've taken some initial steps.

One of the best ways to begin changing your lifestyle and behavior is to take an inventory of how you live your life. The self-test in this chapter will enable you to identify where you are and to what extent everything you've read thus far has changed your lifestyle. You've learned to understand your disease (Step One), learned the importance of and what to expect from your medications (Step Two), learned to eat the right foods and take the right nutraceuticals (Step Three), and learned to commit to and enact an effective exercise program (Step Four). All of this forms a reliable knowledge and activity bank that can help motivate you to make better lifestyle choices.

Studies at the Mayo Clinic and other medical research centers agree that lifestyle change is critical to successful diabetes management. This is often the most challenging aspect of care for both patients and health-care practitioners. Regrettably, many physicians also don't include strong lifestyle modification programs in their treatment plans.

PREPARE YOURSELF FOR LIFESTYLE CHANGE FOR A DIABETIC

Lifestyle change will essentially be the results of your efforts to embrace and enact the recommendations in the first four steps. Just remember that trying to do too much at one time can defeat your entire effort. Since most people with diabetes are balancing medication, food, exercise, and daily responsibilities, trying to affect too much lifestyle change and setting too many goals at once can become self-defeating.

Even small changes will help—and will lead to larger ones.

While the connection of weight loss to improvements in the health of a diabetic was not a surprise to a team of Finnish researchers whose study was published in the *New England Journal of Medicine*, the actual extent of the lifestyle improvement called for to achieve this effect was. "The changes that were required to prevent diabetes were not drastic—they were just modest," said lead study author Jaakko Tuomilehto, M.D., Ph.D., of the National Public

Health Institute. If a person managed to both change his diet and exercise, reduce his calorie intake and improve the quality of his diet, then the effect was the best," he said. "But type 2 diabetes can be prevented by changes in the lifestyles of high-risk subjects . . . Whatever single thing they could do also helped."

According to this study, "People at high risk for developing type 2 diabetes can reduce their chances of getting the disease by 58 percent if they lose as few as ten pounds, exercise, and follow a healthy diet." Keep *that* in mind every time you take a walk around the park.

Here's a true story about a patient with type 2 diabetes whose small change has morphed into more overall changes in his diet choices. At one time, he was an "Oreo junkie" who could consume an entire package in a day. Today, he walks down the snack aisle of the supermarket and literally doesn't notice them. The secret isn't only that he now knows why these snacks are harmful; he has managed to overcome the urge to respond to the trigger (the Oreo package) and reset his brain to seek other snacks. But first he had to understand why he was so attracted to this snack.

In talking with his doctor, he realized that he was a stress junkie, putting in long hours at work and loving it. Stress was his trigger, and he fuelled his stress with sugar and caffeine. He began to change his lifestyle by eliminating sugary foods, which was easier for him than giving up caffeine. While his caffeine load now is only slightly lower, he has made great strides in reducing his stress addiction, reinvented his work behavior, and added simple exercise—mostly walking—to keep stress in check. He's healthier both emotionally and physically.

For people with diabetes, having a goal is good, but making a lifestyle change means permanently reversing negative behaviors. Results count more than anything. Our Oreo addict was successful because he took the process of overcoming his triggers and achieving permanent lifestyle change one step at a time.

PROCLAIM YOUR READINESS TO CHANGE!

According to the American Family Physicians (AFP), proclaiming one's readiness to change is critical to making lifestyle changes. Unfortunately, this declaration can easily become a mantra that does not translate to action, because it is often followed closely by a claim of preparation—"I'm getting ready to. . . ." This can lead to continual rationalizations for postponement. Many people say they are "contemplating" the change their physician recommends or are laying the groundwork for change by reading about diets, asking their friends about exercise programs, or thinking about signing up for one. This is also known as procrastination, and it's frequently due to lack of confidence and a history of failure in achieving goals.

The AFP emphasizes that it's important to recognize and believe the following:

- Healthy eating and increased physical activity can prevent or delay diabetes and its complications. Techniques that facilitate adherence to these lifestyle changes are essential for you to succeed.
- Your readiness to work toward change must be developed gradually. Discuss with your physician any reluctance to change by assessing your conviction and confidence.
- Facing the long-term task of making lifestyle changes benefits from professional assistance, such as the help of doctors or therapists, in setting highly specific behavior-outcome goals and short-term behavior targets.
- You should tailor these goals and targets to your preferences and progress, building your confidence in small steps, and implementing more intensive interventions as you are ready for them.
- At each office visit, your physician's follow-up of your self-monitored activity targets will enhance motivation and allow further customization of your lifestyle change plan.
- A coaching approach can be used to encourage positive choices, develop self-sufficiency, and assist you in identifying and overcoming barriers. Your doctor or nutritionist can play this role.
- A team approach—possibly involving professionals such as a diabetologist, nutritionist, cardiologist, exercise specialist, and/or emotional counselor—will often make a more ambitious set of health objectives that are easier to achieve and easier to stick with.

TAKE A SELF-ASSESSMENT TEST TO MEASURE YOUR CURRENT LIFESTYLE

One good way to get started on a lifestyle program that incorporates what you've learned so far is to take an inventory of your current lifestyle to help identify your first priorities.

Answer the following questions, honestly.

What is your lifestyle like today?_____

_____

Are you a couch potato?_____

_____

Do you have any consistent, weekly exercise routine?_____

_____

Do you park close to stores to avoid walking?_____

_____

How do you spend most of your time at home?_____

_____

How often and where do you eat out?_____

_____

How much alcohol do you drink?_____

_____

Do you smoke? If so, how long have you been smoking and how many cigarettes/packs do you smoke each day?_____

_____

Do you shop smart by reading food labels?_____

_____

Do you keep track of your carb intake?_____

_____

How do you deal with stress?_____

_____

How much sleep do you get?_____

_____

Do you ever "zone out" or nap at work?_____

_____

Are you mentally ready to change?_____

_____

What are your motivations for changing?_____

_____

Are you physically able to achieve your exercise goals?_____

_____

Now assess your inventory. Compare your answers with the discussion points that follow, and then work with your doctor to devise a lifestyle alteration plan. Remember, the goal is permanent lifestyle change, not just weight loss. If you characterize your lifestyle as hectic, overwhelming, or just plain nuts, something is wrong. Your overall goal should be to become physically active. That will clear your head and help you remain calm. Let's talk about each question in turn.

What is your lifestyle like today? Do you basically do the same things you've always done each day and week? Do you feel like you are in a rut? Do you get outside and just take a walk to get some fresh air and restorative light? Do you do anything social or cultural that inspires you? Take a class to improve your skills or just for fun?

An important part of weight loss is having an active life—not a frenetic one but a lifestyle that helps you focus on something other than your weight and diabetes. In short, keep stimulated with friends or a new group you might meet doing something new. You can start by just getting together with a friend or friends to walk at a park.

Are you a couch potato? If you spend more than an hour or two daily lying on the couch and staring at the TV, you will soon be a "baked" couch potato. While it's not likely that your muscles will actually atrophy, the physical mechanisms that you need to activate to increase insulin sensitivity and efficiently use glucose in your blood will be impaired.

Do you have any consistent, weekly exercise routine? The important aspect of this question is whether your exercise is consistent. Establishing a specific time and type of exercise is more likely to work for you than a "fit-it-in" approach. Whether you walk, work out in a gym, or participate in an athletic program, the key is sticking with the program.

Do you park close to stores to avoid walking? Here is a suggestion that really works. When you park several rows away and take those extra steps to the mall entrance someone is watching you, whether it's your family, your children or grandchildren, or the other people who care about you remaining healthy. Every extra step you take will help your health.

How do you spend most of your time at home? What do you do at home to keep active? Do you work in the garden? Do you take on do-it-yourself projects to keep you mentally stimulated?

How often and where do you eat out? Eating out, while watching your diet and balancing your nutritional needs, can be a positive part of your lifestyle. For example, going out once a week or every other week with a friend, partner, or spouse to a good restaurant can be something to look forward to and can lower your stress by enhancing your lifestyle. Having diabetes, needing to lose weight, and watching your health do not mean you have to avoid the fun life. Just keep it under control.

How much alcohol do you drink? Depending on your medical condition and despite the myths about the long-lived French, alcohol doesn't offer a great lifestyle benefit to people with diabetes or cardiovascular disease. There are many closet drinkers, and it's easy to go overboard with it. For people who don't have severe weight problems, a small glass of red wine—not an 8-ounce (235 ml) glass—is acceptable with dinner. In some cases one alcoholic beverage a day is allowed. However, for the people in poor health who most need weight loss, no alcohol intake is advised.

Do you shop smart by reading food labels? The more you learn about the types of foods that lead to the right balance of protein, carbohydrates, and fats in your meals, the easier the rest of your lifestyle changes will be. However, unless you learn how to read and understand the labels on everything you buy, your attempts to change may be derailed. It's not a bad idea to become somewhat compulsive about this. It will help you be more aware of what you are buying.

Do you keep track of your carb intake? Adapt some or all of the meal plans found on pages 100 to 105 in this book as a way to get started.

How do you deal with stress? While you will find an entire chapter on stress reduction later in this book, it's important to consider this as part of your assessment of your current lifestyle. Stress is complicated because it is often both a symptom (panic disorder) and an actual illness that psychiatrists call generalized anxiety disorder. Anxiety and stress can have a devastating effect on you physically and also cripple you emotionally, causing loss of desire to keep going in your diabetes control program. Of all the issues that come up as you try to modify your lifestyle as a diabetic, discuss stress with a professional and treat it promptly. Later we will discuss ways to make stress work for you, but first it has to be under control.

How much sleep do you get? Sleep experts indicate that virtually every American gets too little sleep. In general, people should get at least eight hours, but most rarely get even six to seven hours. Many people also have one of a variety of sleep disorders: snoring, sleep apnea, insomnia, restless leg syndrome, and even sleep disruption caused by some underlying metabolic disorder. Sleep problems cause stress, and they also weaken your immune system and have an overall negative impact on your lifestyle. This is another area of your lifestyle that you should consult a doctor about if necessary; don't resort to any sort of medication or over-the-counter pills that can interact with and compromise your diabetes medications.

Do you ever "zone out" or nap at work? This doesn't have to mean falling asleep at your desk. It might be just that you lose concentration or find yourself nodding off. You might even become dizzy when you stand up quickly. If this happens more than once or twice in a row, it's not because you aren't getting enough sleep. It may mean that your medications aren't working properly or your blood sugar has suddenly dropped.

Are you mentally ready to change? It's vital that you look inside and make sure you are ready to make these lifestyle changes. Setbacks don't equal failure. Think about exercising and try to do it as often as possible until you achieve consistency. Concentrate on learning to buy good foods that eliminate the high levels of carbohydrates you used to consume. To do this, concentrate on going to a supermarket and buying only what you need, not boxes of sweets, at least 90 percent of the time.

Continually "talk" to yourself about the different parts of your life-change plan and make sure the answer to every one of them is yes. If you can't say that you are ready, then make sure you talk to your doctor.

What are your motivations for changing? There is only one correct answer: to lose weight and to stay healthy. Try using tools to remain motivated: Tape pictures of your children or family on your treadmill or on the dashboard of your car with notes reminding you, "Don't park close." Tell yourself that you have lots of clothes in the closet that you can't wear any longer and that you refuse to throw out. Remind yourself that being overweight and diabetic threatens your life, and it also leads to a lot of expensive medication. It doesn't have to be that way. Make sure you have tangible motivation that you can rely on when you begin changing your lifestyle.

Are you physically able to achieve your exercise goals? You won't know until you try, but before you start, discuss your exercise program with your doctor and you'll have a good idea of your fitness level.

TAKE THE NEXT STEP IN LIFESTYLE CHANGE: SET PRIORITIES

Once you have an overview of your current lifestyle, view your answers in the context of your medical conditions and needs and use them to help you to set priorities for lifestyle change.

Priority One: Motivation

Some assessment-and-treatment programs don't motivate people to change their lifestyles. For example, many people resist drug therapy. Often, a patient selects a doctor known as a holistic or integrative physician and is disappointed when he or she is told that medications are necessary. This is especially true when he or she is prescribed one of the new medications to reach lowered blood glucose levels.

From a physician's point of view, what motivates patients who are resistant to treatment is their own personal experience—the deterioration of their own health, and/or complications of diabetes in their family, such as amputations, renal dialysis, and blindness.

When I am trying to motivate patients, I often use my own personal experience. I have a picture of my genetic background: my mother with her eight brothers (two of whom died in their fifties) and other family members who died young with diabetes, obesity, and heart disease. I also show them a picture of myself when I was 325 pounds (147.4 kg). I'm the poster boy.

keep yourself on track

Here are some ways to keep yourself motivated:

- Remember all of the ways diabetes can affect your health and increase your risk for heart disease, hypertension, and other medical problems.
- Remember to take your medications and work with your doctor to maximize their effectiveness.
- Construct an internal belief that certain foods taste as good as Oreos, and you actually will begin to feel better when you select them instead of the cookies.
- Recognize that exercise begins with a few steps—and take a few more every day.

When people are resistant, I try to associate the reason they came to the center with why they need to get started. What was the reason for their first visit? Whatever that might be, it is significant. Some people have musculoskeletal problems and some are developing vision or circulatory problems; those problems can be used to motivate them to act. It's important for patients who resist treatment to know where they stand on the risk scale of arteriosclerosis and coronary disease, and I counsel them accordingly.

There's no real difference between ages or sexes when it comes to the question of who does better with lifestyle changes. It's all about motivation. Sometimes older people have more commitment, especially when they have grandchildren. It's not uncommon for people to say they want to be there for their grandchildren.

Priority Two: Set Your First Goal with Your Doctor

As noted earlier, it's vital that you have a physician whom you like and respect, who is experienced in treating diabetes, and who has a comprehensive treatment program. Ideally, you and your doctor are together for life. You must be comfortable with him or her and feel that you can be honest.

Sit down with your physician and set a goal—in this case, one that can be achieved by changing your lifestyle. (This will be drawn from the first four steps of this plan.) Base the goal on your current physical condition, as determined by the tests outlined in Step Three.

Priority Three: Set Improved Nutritional Goals

As you know by now, nutrition is as important as exercise and medications in controlling diabetes. Step Three of this plan discusses nutrition in depth, as I do in my initial meeting with patients. Just as nutrition is listed as a top priority here, in reality, improving your nutrition is an important part of each day of your life.

Based on your physical exam, cardiovascular testing, and metabolic profile, your doctor will outline a dietary program for you. In my practice, I often refer patients to one of my medical nutritionists, who develop an individualized eating program for them. Almost always, the nutritionists recommend a low-glycemic, low-carbohydrate, Mediterranean-type diet, as described earlier. Patients receive a written explanation of their nutrition program, and at their next meeting with the nutritionist, he or she will again discuss the physical findings. In almost all cases, patients are told to keep a daily food diary, which can be helpful in managing diabetes and weight loss.

Priority Four: Remember That No One Change Is More Important Than the Others

If you had to choose between taking your medications and changing your diet, which would you pick? The choice is not as simple as it seems because compliance is everything in managing diabetes and losing excess weight without causing further impaired glucose tolerance and continued damage to your kidneys, pancreas, and liver. This program is really a commitment. That means you have to continue to work with your doctor in spite of setbacks. Longtime follow-up is extremely important: Many patients who have done well slip back into weight gain and poor glucose management because they don't continue to work with their doctors after some initial success.

All aspects of this program are important: lifestyle changes, diet, exercise, stress reduction, nutraceuticals, pharmaceuticals, and following up with your doctor and his or her staff. Because each factor is equally important to your success, one is not more important than another.

Priority Five: Stop Smoking

How do I deal with patients who smoke? As a heart and blood vessel surgeon, much of the devastation of blood vessels I see is caused by smoking. I tell patients with circulatory problems that before they light their next cigarette, they should ask themselves whether they want the cigarette or their leg.

It's a tough problem. You have to keep on them. Many people don't even say they are smokers unless you ask or look at their history. I consider all treatment options. I have sometimes used outside resources such as smoking cessation programs that have been shown to be successful. I recommend bioenergetics, which is a type of psychotherapy, and I suggest acupuncture. I am also starting to have some good luck with the drug varenicline (brand name Chantix).

Stopping smoking is the single most important thing a smoker can do to help defeat diabetes. Smoking triples your risk of diabetes and diminishes the effect of insulin. Smoking also increases the likelihood for developing neuropathy, kidney disease, cardiovascular damage, and vision loss.

Chapter Five gives some insight and guidance on quitting smoking, which many feel is one of the most difficult lifestyle changes of all.

Priority Six: Make Lifestyle Changes as a Cardio-Diabetes Patient

If you have severe cardiac problems and need to exercise, you must join a monitored cardiac exercise program because you need a more intensive program. If you are developing cardiovascular complications, you need a more intensive diet program, more monitored exercise, and more intense management of your diabetes and lipids. To make a lifestyle change, you must take a comprehensive approach—because of your diabetes, and also because you need to take additional nutraceuticals and drugs to lower your lipids and to treat hypertension, arrhythmia, or poor cardiac function. You need to see a physician who can address both your cardiovascular and nutritional needs.

MAKE YOUR OWN PLAN FOR CHANGE

To control your diabetes and lose weight, you have to construct your own plan for lifestyle change that uses all the tools and support ideas you've learned so far. Admittedly, it's easier to do a lifestyle assessment and set priorities than to actually carry out the plan, yet thousands of people who have taken control of their diabetes and weight loss in this manner have succeeded.

Here are a few of their stories from my practice to give you some more insight.

Judy Takes Control

Judy, the branch manager of a bank, is fifty-five years old. She was recently diagnosed with type 2 diabetes after having prediabetes for several years. Judy is overweight, but not obese, and she does not have a family history of diabetes. During her years with prediabetes, she stuck with her diet and generally took care of herself.

Three years ago, Judy's life fell apart. She was diagnosed with cancer and spent months in treatment. Fortunately, she came through that and felt ready to get back to work and reassume her family responsibilities, which included taking care of her eighty-three-year-old mother, who had vision problems.

Then Judy was diagnosed with a brain tumor, which turned out to be benign, although she developed partial facial paralysis.

Many people might throw in the towel at that point. Not Judy. She says that being diagnosed with diabetes scared her most because untreated diabetes has serious complications, and her bout with cancer caused her to lose focus in her diabetes treatments.

Once Judy was able to get back on track, she began taking a new medication that helped, and she took control of her life in another important way. Using her executive skills, she began to educate herself about her diabetes. She signed up for a number of e-newsletters and began to follow developments every time she saw a new article on diabetes management.

"By educating myself in this way, I was able to understand what I had to do, and it reinforced the things my nutritionist and doctor emphasized," Judy says. "It helped me remember to be aware of my numbers [blood sugar levels] and to take my medications. I've also emphasized fiber in my diet."

Judy reports that she tried branded weight loss programs in the past with little success, and she realizes that a carefully chosen diet and exercise are keys to success. She says that she's able to stay motivated to change. "I've had to learn to make adjustments and not beat myself up," Judy says. "I try to do the best I can."

James Starts Listening

James was one of "New York's finest," a tough cop who retired after thirty years on the force. Over the years, James says he's seen it all. He and his wife, Phyllis, raised three children, sent them to college, and watched them become a nurse, a lawyer, and a dietician.

But within the past fifteen years, James developed diabetes and gained weight until his 5-foot, 8-inch (173 cm) frame carried 240 pounds (109 kg).

"I was always heavy as a cop," James says. "I was eating all garbage: hero sandwiches, take-out food, pasta, cheese, and snacks."

Eventually, James's lifestyle choices, a family history of diabetes, and the stress of his job caught up with him, and James found it hard to catch his breath after mild exertion and started getting staph infections. He saw a number of doctors, who did not help him. James continued to gain weight, eventually reaching more than 250 pounds (114 kg).

At this point, James developed cardiac complications and underwent angioplasty. When blood test results indicated that he needed to start taking insulin and should undergo an invasive heart procedure, he decided to look for an alternative.

"I didn't want surgery or any other open-heart procedure," James says. "When I heard Dr. Vagnini on the radio, I decided to go see him, and between him and Maria Santoro, his nutritionist, I finally began to understand what I needed to do. Then one of my friends passed away, and I had a lot more motivation."

"Now my food intake is totally different, and I've lost 60 pounds (27 kg) in 6 months," James says. "I started listening. That is the real change. I can walk now and get around, but as soon as I put any weight back on, that changes."

James changed his diet from wolfing mammoth portions of junk food to eating small portions of healthy food, such as a can of tuna and vegetables for lunch, and taking supplements that help with weight loss. He admits that he was suspicious at first of the value of taking supplements, but he kept with it. "It really worked," he says.

At home, James does his own thing, including cooking and watching the carbs. "When we go out to eat, I look at the amount of food I eat," James says. "In the beginning, it was hard because I loved dessert, but I was able to stop."

James's medication regimen changed, too. When he began insulin, he says, "I didn't like the needles, having to carry them around wherever I went, but now there are insulin pens, and those are easy to use and very portable."

Now age seventy-two, James walks on a treadmill three times a week, has added some sit-ups, and has begun lifting light weights again.

"This has been a real struggle," says the man who spent decades patrolling dangerous neighborhoods. "But you have to ask, do you want to live or die? Otherwise you'll be down below."

As for handling stress, James was told by Dr. Vagnini to consider saying a prayer, and that's what he does.

Sue Survives Trials of a Thin Diabetic

Sue, fifty-two years old, is a paralegal at a busy law firm. She puts in long hours to keep up with the constant paperwork that keeps her sedentary during the day and exhausted in the evening. She has type 2 diabetes with a strong family history of the disease that stretches back two generations on both sides of the family.

Thin and fit at 5 feet, 4 inches (163 cm) tall and 130 pounds (59 kg), Sue was diagnosed with diabetes at age thirty-nine. "I really didn't know anything, and I was in denial when I first got it," Sue says. "I was very sick, with blood sugars of 450 to 500. I felt horrible, and my first doctors missed my diagnosis."

It turned out that Sue has a problem that affects about 20 percent of people with diabetes, who are sometimes referred to as "thin" diabetics. "I always had low blood sugar as a kid and pretty much ate what I wanted to eat," she recalls.

Thin diabetics—diabetics who are not overweight—frequently have to take insulin, as Sue does now, but they usually are started on oral drugs, such as metformin (brand name Glucophage). Sue was prescribed one of the older drugs that were the only treatments available at that time. "I waited too long to go on insulin," she says.

Unfortunately, when Sue needed to start taking insulin, she was told that she would be taking insulin multiple times a day, as if she had type 1 diabetes. She initially tried to minimize her use of insulin, because she couldn't tolerate the side effects.

The solution for Sue was an insulin pump, which is a device that automatically delivers a measured dose of insulin to the body through a process known as continuous subcutaneous insulin infusion therapy. The device is about the size of a cell phone, and it's carried in a holster on the waist or on another part of the body. It's hooked up to a cannula, which is a sort of permanent tube under the skin. When Sue uses the pump, she simply attaches it to the cannula and goes about her daily activities.

Along with receiving insulin through the insulin pump, Sue counts carbohydrates. Her blood sugars have been normal for more than four years. Like Judy, she educates herself about developments in diabetes management and practices stress-reducing activities such as yoga and biofeedback, which is an alternative form of medicine that enables you to gain control of your emotions by becoming aware of the bodily reactions such as the rise in blood pressure that they invoke. Sue also takes a large number of vitamins and even cod liver oil, which she feels works for her but might not work for you.

Sue attributes her success to her combination approach to managing her diabetes. "One [component] does not work without the others," she says. "I walk on the treadmill, and I go for regular checkups, but it has not been easy. When I was younger, I ate whatever I wanted because I came from a thin family, which turned out to be a family of thin diabetics. I had to give up certain foods that I really liked."

"In the morning, I eat bread that is a dense grain with no yeast. Sometimes I have cinnamon raisin bread with cashew or peanut butter to slow absorption of sugar. Lunch is tuna or egg salad on dense bread or a Caesar salad without croutons and perhaps a small piece of fruit," she explains. "Dinner might be a very large salad with small amounts of protein, but I don't keep much food in the house."

Sue feels she's "done great," has a lot of tools for managing her diabetes, and feels better than she did fifteen years ago. People tell her she looks great, too.

"These tools are part of my motivation, and exercise is my number-one tool," she says.

Albert Becomes a Determined Dieter

Albert is sixty-six years old, 6 feet, 1 inch (185 cm) tall, and weighs more than 270 pounds (122 kg). Two years ago, he retired from an academic position at a local college, looking forward to a relaxed retirement with his wife and grandchildren. While Albert has a family history of diabetes, it is limited to his parents, who both developed the disease late in life.

Albert developed diabetes and has required insulin for the past nineteen years. Albert struggles to get his weight down to 200 pounds (91 kg) and recently has been diagnosed with heart problems. At one point, he was admitted to the hospital with suspected congestive heart failure, which turned out not to be the case. He has experienced cardiac arrhythmia and elevated blood pressure, and he takes diuretics and blood pressure medication. Albert also suffers from sleep apnea and uses a special breathing device while sleeping.

Albert is in a position many people with diabetes find themselves in: taking multiple pills for various disorders along with insulin shots and following a specific diet. His weight fluctuation caused one of his doctors to suggest gastric bypass surgery, which is something Albert has rejected out of hand. But this has motivated him to try to gain control of his diabetes on his own. Since Albert has a bad back, he has problems when he exercises, so his current focus is in managing his weight through diet.

"I try to keep on a steady diet," Albert says. "I don't eat cakes and things like that, and I really want to get back to 200 pounds (91 kg). Most of my meals include a protein, a larger portion of a green vegetable, and maybe a small portion of pasta or potatoes on the side. We don't eat out often—maybe once every two weeks."

Like Judy, Sue, and James, Albert constantly searches for information to help him manage his disease. "I'm very facile with a computer, and I'm always looking up information to expand on what I read in the newspaper or magazines," he says. "I've even found some new drug trials that I'm following to see if these medications are a possibility for me."

Albert says that one thing has helped him substantially. "[Retiring] was the best way I have found to relieve stress!"

MAKE A GAME PLAN

Now that you've read all five steps of this plan, fill in the following form. Then in the next chapter, you'll see how this information comes together for your health and weight loss needs.

Are you ready to start?_____

_____

What is your first priority going to be?_____

_____

What is your specific goal, including exactly when you will start?_____

_____

What are the roadblocks to your goal?_____

_____

How can you overcome these roadblocks?_____

_____

Do you have a support group set up?_____

_____

What will you add to your program next?_____

_____

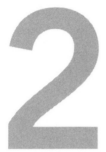

Learn How All Five Steps Work Together to Help You Lose Weight

THE SECRET TO THIS PLAN

Over the last several pages, you have been presented with plate after plate of information. You aren't expected to learn or memorize it all, but over time you will integrate it into your life simply because you will feel better as you do it.

The question you still might want answered, however, is: Is all of this really going to help me lose weight?

The answer is, absolutely.

Okay—how?

At the beginning of this book, I said that weight loss is always going to be the main benefit of the Five-Step Plan. You begin with education, then your medications must be chosen carefully and working properly, and your nutritional choices as outlined need to be followed with exercise and other lifestyle changes. However, there is one more big, extra benefit. When all five come together, the biological combination enables your insulin sensitivity to increase and weight loss will automatically follow. You are optimizing every part of your body and environment that contributes to weight loss.

Here are two ways to look at it. First, imagine that you are a talented young violinist who practices many hours a day and plays in a string quartet for a few years in high school. When you go to an advanced music school, you discover that you can do more. After several years, you go to a tryout and become a member of a large, successful orchestra.

On opening night, everyone is dressed in their tuxedos, and you take your place, as the conductor steps out and raises his baton. On the downbeat, you all begin to play. Suddenly you realize that your individual skill and that of the brass section, the woodwinds, the rest of the strings, and percussion have done something amazing. You are all excellent individual musicians, but together you have created the sound necessary to perform a symphony!

Second, many men and women have played softball or baseball in their youth—pickup games or youth leagues where you chose sides and just had fun. If you happened to be a very good ball player, you might make it to the "Bigs" and play professionally. Some athletes get that far but don't become stars, lasting only a few seasons, while others become superstars.

The reason is that the superstars can optimize their many skills. They can get a base hit when they have to or smash a bases-loaded homer to win a game. They are talented at offense and defense; they make dramatic diving catches in the outfield, steal bases, lay down a perfect bunt, hit to the opposite field, and throw out the runner at home plate from their knees!

These two scenarios are perfect examples of why learning to integrate all of the five steps into your life will bring weight loss. As you do this, you will crush the roadblocks described in each chapter and make yourself into a multifaceted person, a superstar who can do it all.

Another common thread runs through these examples and your enactment of the Five-Step Plan: It takes lots of concerted and sustained effort to get to the top—to succeed, or in your case to lose weight. You need to make that effort to break through the roadblocks, because your life is at stake.

One way to make this easier is to remember that as you absorb the information and make certain changes—such as changing your food plan for a month—they will all become part of a chain reaction that will start toppling the roadblocks.

If, over time, you can accomplish what is recommended in Steps 1 through 6, then you will become an MVP—your personal team's most valuable player!

KNOW HOW LONG IT TAKES TO FEEL AN EFFECT

If you study the steps, initiate them properly, and stick to it, you will begin losing weight and bring your glucose numbers into control within the first two or three weeks. It is very important that you continue taking your medications (Step Two) as prescribed and keep track of your blood glucose levels daily, reporting any problems to your physician or nutritionist.

To keep you motivated and remind you of how different this process is from other so-called diets, keep the following points in mind.

This is a healthy diet. You might think that a healthy diet means nothing but tofu and soy burgers, but the opposite is true. You'll select from a wide range of foods combined in the proper proportions and in reasonable amounts. If you have cardiovascular complications, you'll incorporate low-fat foods into your meals to control or reduce plaque buildup in your arteries.

Stop counting calories. This plan does not involve counting calories, but you have to be aware of your overall caloric consumption. A calorie is just a number. You won't have to count calories because you will not crave calorie-rich foods, and your body will burn the carbs you do eat to produce energy.

Anyone can use this plan. This meal/weight loss plan does not exclude vegetarians or meat-and-potato eaters because it provides proteins and fiber that help you meet daily nutritional needs.

This plan protects against sudden drops in blood sugar. This is one of the scariest aspects of diabetes. Most people are unprepared for it, and they have to scramble for some sugar or juice. This diet is likely to reduce that risk significantly.

This plan satisfies your appetite. You'll stop bingeing and craving food because you'll be eating protein and "good" carbs and fiber.

You'll avoid carbo-drift. After losing weight, you won't be tempted to drift back into your old eating habits.

This plan avoids the dangers of too-rapid weight loss. Experts agree that rapidly dropping pounds simply leads to the "yo-yo" effect (losing and then gaining back from continual attempts at dieting). You'll make a real change by making proper eating choices for successful long-term weight maintenance.

Clear medical benefits will occur that will also be reflected by the thinner you in the mirror. These benefits are explained in the following list:

- You will intensify your body's ability to generate energy by raising your metabolic rate through the food choices you make. Protein boosts thermogenesis for weight loss, while excess carbohydrate intake slows your ability to burn fat.
- You will control inflammation by avoiding saturated-fat-filled foods, sugar, and other dietary fats. Inflammatory disease is a significant aspect of obesity and diabetes. It accelerates the aging process, and it also adds to the multiple detrimental physiological diseases that might already be present. It puts you at risk for chronic disease, contributes to heartburn, and makes it more difficult to control glucose and insulin levels.
- You will reduce beta cell stress syndrome, gastrointestinal complications (such as gas and bloating), excess water in the body, food allergies, and gluten intolerance with weight loss.
- You will consume higher levels of fiber which will help you detoxify, control glucose and insulin levels, and reduce weight and inflammation.

Ultimately your meal plan is determined by you, based on the following:

- Your level of diabetes, as defined by your overall blood glucose levels measured in your laboratory-tested blood values, such as hemoglobin A1C, home glucose monitoring, and other factors that include triglycerides, energy levels, and waist size
- Your general health and weight loss needs, as determined by you and your nutritionist
- Your motivation and commitment
- A dietary program of low-carbohydrate meals based your individual situation
- Drug therapy, nutraceuticals, vitamins, and other weight-reducing supplements that have been tested and used successfully at the New York Heart, Diabetes and Weight Loss Center. (The nutraceuticals program is described in Step Three.)

In the following chapters, we will take a look at some more roadblocks that can keep you from losing weight. These are what some people call behavioral roadblocks, and they include the effect of stress and sleep deprivation. Adding them to the information and recommendations in the previous chapters will eliminate negative aspects of your life that can keep you on the sidelines or sliding backward in your efforts to eat right, exercise, and take your medications.

**PART TWO: LIVING AND LOSING WEIGHT
IN THE REAL WORLD**

Sometimes losing weight loss is complicated for a diabetic: You have continued to stay overweight despite your best efforts to follow the medically based recommendations in this book.

You may be missing another, often overlooked roadblock: You live in the real world, where everyday life can increase your risk of diabetes and thwart weight loss success. In spite of your efforts to turn around your lifestyle (see Step Five) and follow all of the other steps in this plan faithfully, things you do every day may unconsciously increase your chances of developing diabetes and other complications.

A few years ago, a popular Ricky Martin song, "Livin' La Vida Loca" (the Crazy Life) warned what could happen if certain things in life get out of hand. It's a good warning for people who have been procrastinating and resisting change where their health is concerned. While few people go to the lifestyle extremes described in the song, resisting losing weight, increasing blood glucose levels, and raising your risk for heart disease adds up to a level of the "la vida loca" that can put you on the precipice of health disasters.

Gaining control of your physical and mental health makes the difference in whether your prediabetes or type 2 diabetes reaches a crisis. In the following short chapters, you can take a closer look at the following real-world issues that can confound your weight loss and diabetes control goals and learn strategies that can help you get past these roadblocks:

- The special problems that women face with diabetes and weight loss
- Smoking cessation
- Stress and depression
- Sleep problems
- Building family support

You might have many of these challenges in your life right now. You cannot cope with all of these problems at once, and you might not be able to handle them alone, but the effort you invest in managing the effect of these factors in your life will pay off in heading off your close encounter with "la vida loca."

The key is to face each of these roadblocks and take a single step at a time to overcome it.

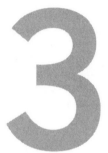

3

Women, Diabetes, and Weight Loss

THE TRIPLE CHALLENGE

Weight control is a critical health issue for women today. In the United States, 50 percent of women between the ages of twenty and seventy-four are now overweight or obese, which is a problem shared by their sisters around the world. According to a 2002 Centers for Disease Control and Prevention (CDC) report, the average American woman between the ages of eighteen and seventy-four stands 5 feet, 4 inches (163 cm) tall and weighs 164 pounds (74 kg), nearly 25 pounds (11 kg) heavier than the average American woman in the 1960s.

Today, the female population is living longer than ever and, with that, the natural incidence of type 2 diabetes is growing.

The Five-Step Plan is particularly valuable to women who are obese and not just because of the clear risks for diabetes. Without adopting every one of the steps, a woman with diabetes has an even less chance than a man with diabetes of reducing weight. One reason is that a woman's metabolic system is different than a man's. Women tend to accumulate fat differently, in different places on their bodies—fat that is more difficult to burn off without increased exercise as in Step Four. Research conducted at Mt. Sinai Hospital Medical School in New York suggests women are more susceptible to the lures of overeating. Actual changes in the brains of men and women were measured when food was present, and then removed. In women, temptation and desire for the food was more powerful when it was present, and lasted longer after it was gone.

More than ever before, women need to focus on losing weight by learning more about the specific roadblocks that can make weight loss more difficult for them and what they can do about it.

UNDERSTAND WHY SOME WOMEN GAIN WEIGHT— DESPITE THEIR BEST EFFORTS

For decades, women have been assaulted by messages and images that suggest—and not subtly—that if they look a certain way, they will be healthy and happy. In other words, lose weight, be thin, and be on the cover of a fashion magazine. This is how the ultimate body image goal for women is too often pitched. As a result, women spend billions of dollars to drop pounds that inevitably return.

Why do so many weight loss programs for women fail in the long run? It's not for lack of trying. It's not uncommon for a woman to spend upward of $10,000 in a few years and try as many as ten different systems. According to Karen Chalmers, M.S., R.D., director of nutrition at the famed Joslin Diabetes Center in Boston, women today are the first of the "Weight Watchers Generation."

Often women are on multiple medications and might be tempted to try over-the-counter weight loss products that can interact with them. Plus, of course, obesity leads to an inactive lifestyle. Most important of all, women are often caught in the "meal trap," trying to feed various family members who demand food now or eat a seemingly continual meal including snacks and desserts, adding to the temptations.

RESIST A RISKY SHORTCUT

Chalmers talked to many different groups of women who required insulin for their diabetes and found a common factor in their weight loss attempts: insulin manipulation. As mentioned earlier, many people believe that insulin leads to weight gain and decide to reduce their insulin dosage without the knowledge of their physician. They soon find that a few pounds melt off quickly, then return when they resume their normal dose of insulin. This, Chalmers notes, is a "risky balancing act."

When the level of insulin is reduced, blood sugar levels rise, which in turn leads to dehydration from fluid loss. When you resume the regular dosage, hunger increases as the body quickly consumes the insulin, you retain fluid, and your glucose goes up. Each time you self-treat, your insulin level responds in yo-yo fashion. Along with self-medicating like this, many people skip meals or follow branded diets that are fine for overweight people without diabetes, but that send the diabetic's metabolism into a tailspin. With recurrent attempts to diet and lose weight, you might actually end up with a chronic metabolic slowdown.

While branded weight loss programs work for some people, weight loss and weight management in people with diabetes can only be achieved by confronting and overcoming the biological roadblocks outlined in previous chapters. The only diet and medication regimen that works for people with diabetes is one that is tailored by the doctor to your situation, described in the five steps in this book.

Despite the pressures of the "thin culture," it's important to understand that the goal of weight loss in women is to achieve metabolic fitness, which may be at a weight where you might not necessarily be thin, but at which your lipids and glucose levels are correct and you have achieved some level of physical fitness.

AVOID CARDIOVASCULAR DISEASE

Women face biological and sociological health issues at various stages in life that are different from those of men, and many of these only underline the importance of weight loss.

Of all the health issues related to diabetes that face women today, heart disease, especially coronary artery disease—is the most threatening. Diabetes has always been a top risk factor for cardiovascular disease in both sexes, but today it's likely that every woman over age fifty is at risk for heart disease, and 25 percent may die from it. Coronary heart disease is the number-one killer of women over age twenty-five. According to the American Heart Association (AHA), one in three women who died suddenly from heart disease showed no previous symptoms and might not even have known that they had prediabetes. One-third of women with high blood pressure have been found to have prediabetes or type 2 diabetes.

One in 2.6 women die from heart disease, compared with 1 in 30 from breast cancer. Heart disease claims more women's lives than the next four most common causes of female death combined. While education and women's greater awareness of how to better use the health-care system (making sure they attend to health issues beyond the gynecological) are beginning to improve the odds, the risks of diabetes and coronary artery disease remain elevated as long as their weight level remains high. According to Michael L. Dansinger, M.D., "As long as pounds are lost, heart risk goes down. Losing 20 pounds (9 kg) corresponds to about 30 percent reduction in heart risk score." However, this does not necessarily mean that the risk of heart attack also is reduced.

For many years, only ob-gyns were particularly aware of the potential for heart disease among obese women, but they seldom checked for elevated glucose levels at their yearly exam. Even today, fewer than 20 percent of physicians recognize that more women than men die of heart disease. Fortunately, many physicians now are becoming more aware of the risks to women from weight gain and diabetes, but you still have to be educated and communicate with your physician, particularly if you have a family history of heart disease or diabetes.

Connecting Female Hormones and Heart Disease

Another reason women become victims of heart disease despite the growing body of information on the connection between diabetes and obesity, is a sort of biological half-myth that is really a roadblock because it can keep someone from seeking early diagnosis. For years many people, women and health professionals as well, believed that estrogen, a naturally occurring hormone produced in women until menopause, offered women special protection from developing heart disease and diabetes. Many ongoing studies have concluded that estrogen affects many organ systems in women, ranging from influencing the creation of blood clots to helping to regulate blood pressure.

Other studies have shown that at menopause when estrogen levels drop, women become more insulin resistant, and start gaining weight. Women's risk for heart disease, in general, is lower prior to the onset of menopause. After menopause, studies have shown that the risk of heart disease rises slowly until age sixty-five, when risks for heart attack between men and women evens out; this catches many women and their doctors by surprise.

Why does estrogen help protect women from heart disease? Estrogen has a positive effect on HDL, the "good" cholesterol, and a lowering effect on LDL, the "bad" cholesterol. Plus, estrogen can help lower overall total cholesterol.

So it is partially true that estrogen is the reason that women have usually developed heart disease at a later age than do men. Women have lower risk at the same age as when men's symptoms of heart disease begin to appear. However, this is beginning to change as risk factors including smoking and stress are being recognized as significant in women and more accurate and earlier diagnoses are made.

Considering Hormone Replacement Therapy

Many women who are approaching or experiencing menopause have been confused about the protection from heart disease provided by hormone replacement therapy (HRT). In the early 1990s, synthetic estrogen (brand name Premarin) was widely prescribed for relief of menopause symptoms until several large studies linked HRT with increased risk of heart attack.

By late 2004, some conclusions were finally reached about the use of HRT among postmenopausal women and how it relates to heart and stroke risk. The AHA and the U.S. Food and Drug Administration have published official guidelines that indicate the following:

- HRT is not for heart attack prevention. It does not replace the natural estrogen that protects younger women.
- At times, HRT has been prescribed for other uses, such as prevention of bone disease. However, the benefits and the risks are not proven.
- Women currently at risk for heart disease or with heart disease should not use HRT without a physician's specific approval.
- HRT is a good method of reducing postmenopausal symptoms over a short period.
- HRT does not prevent heart disease with long-term use.

bio-identical hormone therapy

In my practice, I prescribe bio-identical hormone therapy. This is a form of hormone replacement championed by actress Suzanne Somers. You purchase it from a compounding pharmacist, and it's a more natural approach than the pharmacologic replacement therapy. I've found this an important adjunct to the weight loss program of my menopausal women patients.

An important point to remember when considering the controversy is that hundreds of thousands of women use HRT every day and have done so for years. Clearly, this is a question between you and your physician. However, there seems to be very little question that once you hit menopause, the natural biological advantage of reduced risk of heart disease that you have as a woman is no longer present, rather the risk is increased with weight, diabetes, and insulin resistance.

An important note about oral contraceptives: Most oral contraceptives containing estrogen have been shown to increase heart disease and diabetes risks by increasing blood glucose levels and making glucose control more difficult. Oral contraceptives have also been linked to blood clots. The risks of oral contraceptive use are well documented.

These risks are increased if you smoke. If you smoke, quit, especially if you take oral contraceptives and have diabetes.

WATCH FOR CARDIOVASCULAR DISEASE SYMPTOMS

You might not be surprised to read that the symptoms of cardiovascular disease are different in women than in men. One of the most important developments in cardiac treatment over the past decade is increased aware-ness of the similarities and differences in cardiovascular symptoms and risk factors in men and women. Unfortunately, many women with lipid problems and high blood pressure have an underlying glucose problem that can lead to diabetes and heart disease, in other words, the glucose–heart disease connection. For this reason, women have to be doubly vigilant about their weight because of the association between weight gain and heart disease.

About ten years ago, the National Institutes of Health (NIH) initiated the Women's Ischemia Syndrome Evaluation Study (WISE) to assess this threat and to seek new ways to treat women after a more accurate diagnosis is made. The study found surprising results. In as many as three million U.S. women with coronary heart disease, cholesterol plaque may not build up into major blockages, but, instead, spreads evenly throughout the artery wall. As a result, diagnostic coronary angiography reveals that these women have "clear" arteries—no blockages—incorrectly indicating low risk. Despite this, many of these women have a high risk for heart attack. This condition was labeled coronary microvascular syndrome, also called Syndrome X. Syndrome X is not a metabolic syndrome. Syndrome X is characterized by elevated insulin levels; metabolic syndrome is characterized by coronary artery complications, elevated lipid levels, and hypertension.

This confusion is yet another prime example of why risk for women is often missed. In microvascular syndrome, according to the NIH, plaque accumulates in very small arteries of the heart, causing narrowing, reduced oxygen flow to the heart, and pain that can be similar to that of people with blocked arteries, but the plaque does not show up when physicians use standard tests.

WISE investigators found that the majority of women with "clear" angiography who are not diagnosed will continue to have symptoms, declining quality of life, and repeated hospitalizations and tests.

"When a diagnosis of this condition is missed, women are not treated for their angina and high cholesterol, and they remain at high risk for having a heart attack," says National Heart, Lung, and Blood Institute (NHLBI) director Elizabeth G. Nabel, M.D. "This study and the high prevalence of coronary microvascular dysfunction demonstrate that we must think out of the box when it comes to the evaluation and diagnosis of heart disease in women."

Diabetes is a major risk factor for heart disease in men and women. However, if the symptoms are as unclear as this study shows, a woman may find that she is only being treated for her diabetes until her heart disease becomes life threatening.

Other physical ailments—including shortness of breath without chest pain, chills, cold sweats, nausea, light-headedness, palpitations, sleeping and anxiety problems—may or may not be related to heart disease. They are frequently ascribed to other ailments or dismissed altogether.

Many women experience the same heart attack symptoms as men: chest pain, angina, severe pressure in the chest that comes and goes, pain extending down the left arm, pain in the neck or jaw, and sudden exhaustion. Many people liken the pressure or pain in the chest to severe indigestion or heartburn. However, women often do not experience chest pain.

Treating Heart Disease in Women

Abundant information is available on heart disease in women. Groups such as the AHA, American Diabetes Association, and medical institutions are focused on research leading to more effective medication and surgical solutions. Beyond the issues of hormone replacement therapy, treatment of women for heart disease may also differ from treatment of men because women are built on a smaller scale than men. The heart is smaller, and so are the arteries, which can make angioplasty more difficult. Several other factors may enter into treatment for women; however, the same arsenal of education, behavior modification, medication, and exercise is still the front-line defense.

A significant number of women remain at great risk because they are not focused on weight loss. The number-one preventive measure is weight loss.

According to the Society for Women's Health Research, because weight gain and fat deposits differ between women and men, research into these differences can generate tremendous information about the development and progression of heart disease. Fat distribution and body shape are different in men and women. Adipose tissue, present in both men and women, stores fat and is drawn on to supply energy. However, distribution of adipose fat is different between men and women, which may play a role in cardio-vascular risk.

Reducing Cardiovascular Disease in Women

In the past decade, with the increase in heart disease (and death from it) in women, the understanding of clinical issues in women and heart disease, and the initiation of Go Red For Women (a heart disease awareness movement), there has been a greater understanding of the differences that have to be considered when a patient is evaluated and diagnosed.

In February, 2007, the AHA issued further important recommendations for women age twenty and over. "Guidelines for Preventing Cardiovascular Disease in Women," which was published in a special women's health issue of *Circula-*

tion: Journal of the American Heart Association, addressed important subjects, such as aspirin use, mineral supplements, hormone therapy, and stroke prevention.

The AHA's guidelines were also significant because they were reviewed by experts in the fields of cardiology, epidemiology, family medicine, gynecology, internal medicine, neurology, nursing, public health, statistics, and surgery.

"The updated guidelines emphasize the lifetime risks of women, not just the more short-term focus of the 2004 guidelines," said Lori Mosca, M.D., Ph.D., director of preventive cardiology at New York–Presbyterian Hospital and chair of the AHA expert panel that wrote the guidelines. "We took a long-term view of heart disease prevention because the lifetime risk of dying of cardiovascular disease is nearly one in three for women. This underscores the importance of healthy lifestyles in women of all ages to reduce the long-term risk of heart and blood vessel diseases."

The reason education for women is important is because they seem to defer to the health needs of their spouses or partners. When men are asked why they are in the doctor's office, at least 50 percent respond, "My wife made me come." Physicians should take advantage of this moment to bring the wife or female partner into the equation and discuss her health risks. If you are making a doctor's appointment for your spouse, make one for yourself, too!

KEEPING SPECIAL POPULATIONS IN MIND

One overlooked aspect of diabetes management in women has been access to care for many special populations, which includes minority ethnic groups and the uninsured. Many of these women suffer from multiple conditions, especially diabetes, because of genetic risk and poor diet.

The CDC reports that the face of the American female population is changing. Within several decades, 25 percent of women in the United States will be of Hispanic heritage, 12 percent will be African American, and 1 percent will be Native American. Non-Hispanic Whites will represent only 50 percent of the female population by 2050.

Diabetes is two to four times more common in women of color, a situation the CDC says could reach unimaginable dimensions. The impact of diabetes on the U.S. health-care system is well past the $50 billion mark and is growing by at least 10 percent per decade. There is no question of the association between lower socioeconomic status and diabetes. If you are poor, you likely have to choose between seeking medical care, especially preventive care, and putting food on the table. In this case, access to care might be in an emergency room instead of a seeing a specialist, and nutrition may be the cheapest available: fast food.

The lack of insurance is a major risk factor for early morbidity. However, for women who must take care of children and who have limited access to medical care, the risk of diabetes is far higher than it is in other groups, and it should be a focus of our medical-care system.

KNOW ABOUT OTHER SPECIAL DANGERS OF DIABETES FOR WOMEN

Stroke can strike women more often. The risk of cerebrovascular disease and stroke is actually higher in women than in men and is rising at the same rate as heart disease. A study sponsored by the CDC, the Nurses' Health Study, showed that risk of non-fatal stroke was four times higher among women with diabetes than women without diabetes. Risk of fatal strokes also was higher in women with diabetes.

In fact, women with diabetes are at higher risk for cerebrovascular disease or disorders of the brain caused by high blood pressure. Overweight women with diabetes also are at higher risk for higher levels of LDL "bad" cholesterol.

Another distinctive risk for women is diabetic ketoacidosis (DKA), which is also known as diabetic coma. Women with diabetes are 50 percent more likely than men with diabetes to develop DKA. If your diabetes is uncontrolled or badly managed, you are likely to have high blood glucose levels and a high level of ketones (a by-product of fat metabolism in the blood), which is common in type 1 diabetes. Before synthetic insulin became available, most people with diabetes succumbed to DKA. Lack of problem glucose control and insulin levels are bio-roadblocks to weight loss, and yet another life-threatening condition that women have to be particularly aware of.

Here's one thing that women have working strongly in their favor: Women, in general, are more open to seeing doctors because they usually have dealings with the health-care system at a young age, beginning at puberty. It's important for women to realize, however, that they are not simply at risk for ob-gyn problems, but they are also at greater risk for diabetes and cardiovascular disease. Weight loss, which can be achieved by this book's plan, is the place to start.

what can women do to reduce the effect of diabetes?

For many women with diabetes, risk factors add up faster than in men because often more is expected of women in the workplace in addition to the common responsibilities of taking care of a home and family.

If you have any of the following risk factors, you should consult a diabetologist or a cardiologist or discuss them with your primary care physician:

Family history: Your internist, ob-gyn, and your dentist should be made aware if you have a family history of heart disease.

Elevated total cholesterol and other lipids: Low HDL and high LDL and triglycerides are risk factors and symptoms. Diet is only one way to control elevated lipids. Many effective, proven medications can help to bring high cholesterol under control quickly.

High blood pressure: Also know as hypertension, high blood pressure and diabetes often accompany heart disease and raise risks. Both can be controlled through medication, diet, and exercise.

Stress, depression, and other emotional factors: These are also frequently listed as risk factors for heart attack and heart disease.

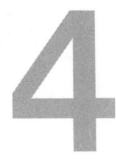

Stress, Diabetes, and Weight Loss

Stress levels across the country have increased in the past several years. As Americans have had to face the deepening financial crisis and other world problems, virtually everyone feels a sense of uneasiness, or free-floating anxiety, every day. With many people wondering if their jobs—and health insurance—will still be there when they go to work, stress levels keep rising. Jobs where people have worked for decades disappear overnight, often leaving those in the age group where chronic disease typically appears without employment and without insurance—yet another roadblock. Even if you have not been affected personally, or only moderately, the continual coverage and frightening reports are enough to make anyone a walking panic attack.

Like many other risk factors that may contribute to diabetes or heart disease, we are now exposed to far more stressors than previous generations have been. We put in far more hours at high-stress jobs than in the past, and this is particularly true for people who define success in terms of how hard we work, how many awards we get, and who becomes the last man standing at a job.

stress stats

- 25 to 40 percent of U.S. workers experience workplace burnout from stress.
- Stress costs U.S. companies up to $300 billion per year in lost productivity, health-related problems, and absenteeism.
- Medical expenses are twice as high for employees who are stressed than for nonstressed workers.
- Depression, frequently accompanied by stress, is the leading occupational disease of this century, responsible for more lost workdays than any other factor.

Negative health consequences attributed to stress include diabetes, heart disease, cancer from smoking, obesity from compulsive eating, liver disease from alcoholism, immunodeficiency, chronic headaches, ulcers, colitis, phobias, panic disorders, and suicide.

Stress is everywhere, and costs the U.S. health-care system billions of dollars each year.

UNDERSTAND THE STRESS–DIABETES– WEIGHT LOSS CONNECTION

The connection between stress, diabetes, and weight loss is a tangled web because stress is a situation caused by both external circumstances and your own biological reactions to them. Stress is linked to diabetes control, and then to weight loss, for the following reasons:

- Stress is often diverting and overwhelming. You lose focus on other important goals in your life.
- Stress can directly cause disease such as high blood pressure and heart disease, which, in turn, affect your diabetes.
- Food behavior is one of the most common responses to stress, frequently leading to extremely bad eating habits as opposed to the dietary program in Step Three. Often stress leads to high-calorie "comfort food" diets, full of sweets and carbohydrates, that can compromise other biological functions because you are not getting enough needed vitamins and other nutrients.

- Stress leads many people with diabetes to fad diets in an effort to feel better about themselves. These usually fail, they gain back anything they've lost, and their stress and weight reach even higher levels.
- Stress can increase smoking and drinking, both of which are diabetes roadblocks. Substituting cigarettes for healthy exercise and high-carb booze for good food may affect weight loss among people with diabetes.

According to Redford Williams, M.D., professor of psychiatry and behavioral sciences at Duke University, Durham, North Carolina, during hard economic times, smokers are 13 percent less likely to quit, and ex-smokers are more likely to relapse. Similarly, when exposed to chronic stress, drinkers tend to drink more, which drives up blood pressure, and alcoholics who have quit drinking are more prone to relapse.

ASSESS YOUR STRESS

Stress is a response to events in your environment, and it's not necessarily or always a negative thing. However, if you experience any of these symptoms randomly, your response to stressful situations in your environment is under-cutting your ability to cope with them. Here are some common symptoms, according to the Cleveland Clinic Stress Management Program:
- Not feeling like yourself
- Feeling overwhelmed
- Being unable to handle workloads that previously had been easy
- Uncalled-for anger, irritability, and tension
- Headaches and tension in your muscles, jaw, or back
- Inability to concentrate or to remember things
- Stomach pain or nausea
- Unusual sweating
- Heart palpitations or rapid heartbeat
- Lack of energy and general disinterest
- Insomnia
- Drinking or using drugs to avoid or block out problems
- Impulsiveness
- Lack of attentiveness
- Obsessive thoughts

- Bad judgment
- Depression and anxiety

Sound familiar? Coping begins with recognizing the problem, understanding it, and formulating a plan to resolve it.

As a diabetic, you need to confront your stress. Jot down your top five stressors as the first step to awareness of just how much stress you have in your life.

1. _____

2. _____

3. _____

4. _____

5. _____

If you experience more than two or three of these situations regularly, you must learn to reduce and manage your stress, perhaps with professional help.

are you a stress junkie?

Many people thrive on stress, setting absurd goals and deadlines and driving themselves to achieve them. We all know people who either love stress or who like to create it at home or in the workplace. In effect, what happens is that stress reinforces itself—you create more to keep on the fast track or to just keep up. Stress junkies should seek professional help and recognize that this lifestyle is going to eventually lead to a crash—either into a wall or over the cliff. Living with someone who is overstressed can be a nightmare, so the most important thing to do in that case is to not become an enabler for that person. Bring the problem out into the open and determine whether or not the stressors can be alleviated or divided. Bring the family into the process.

Stress can increase slowly, building up and leading a catastrophic event. Nip it before it gets you or someone you love.

UNDERSTAND THE CHEMISTRY OF STRESS

The biology of stress is a response that dates back to our days as cave dwellers. When we encounter a potential physical or emotional threat, the body sends a question to the brain via the sympathetic nerves: Do we stand and confront this or turn and head for safety? The feeling of fright sends a signal over the sympathetic nerve system to the adrenal glands, two organs above our kidneys. The brain's signal to the adrenal glands calls for a jolt of adrenalin for energy, endorphins, and cortisol. Once adrenalin is circulating in your body, respiration accelerates, pupils dilate, and you perspire.

If you have diabetes or heart disease, the level of these chemicals in your bloodstream can add strain to an already compromised body. According to the American Diabetes Association (ADA), stress can alter your blood glucose levels in several ways. First, people under stress may not take good care of themselves. They may drink more alcohol or exercise less. They may forget, or not make time, to check their glucose levels or to plan good meals. Second, stress hormones may also alter blood glucose levels directly.

Scientists have studied the effects of stress on glucose levels in animals and people. While most people's glucose levels go up with mental stress, others' glucose levels can go down. In people with type 2 diabetes, mental stress often raises blood glucose levels. Physical stress, such as illness or injury, exacerbates higher blood glucose levels in people with either type 1 or type 2 diabetes.

chart your stress

According to the American Diabetes Association, it's easy to find out whether mental stress affects your glucose control. Before checking your glucose levels, write down a number rating your mental stress level on a scale of one to ten. Then write down your glucose level next to it. After a week or two, look for a pattern. Drawing a graph may help you see trends better. Do high stress levels often occur with high glucose levels, and low stress levels with low glucose levels? If so, stress may affect your glucose control.

If you and your body are constantly facing fight-or-flight moments, you are experiencing adrenal fatigue, and the process can become overwhelming and habitual. Instead of controlling the situation, your body goes into overdrive whenever you face ordinary stressful situations (chronic stress), a vicious circle that can quickly compromise your health.

UNDERSTAND WHAT PROVOKES STRESS

While many environmental, workplace, or personal experiences can create stress, each person tolerates different degrees of stress and responds uniquely. The ADA notes that that some people with type 2 diabetes may also be more sensitive to some of the stress hormones. Relaxing can help by blunting this sensitivity.

Some physicians describe the causes of stress as triggers. You might call them hot buttons, stressors, or pet peeves, but they detonate the brain's fight-or-flight response, and adrenalin, endorphin, cortisol, and blood glucose levels rise and flood your receptors.

CONTROL STRESS

Stress management ideas and advice are everywhere. A Google search produces millions of links to advice pages, counseling services, yoga programs, and products for coping with the stresses of your family and job. For most healthy people, stress management programs make sense. However, people with diabetes should approach stress as an enemy to be eliminated. In addition to the normal array of stressors, diabetes adds the additional stresses of coping with high blood glucose levels, obesity, and cardiovascular complications that limit exercise, so many stress management programs won't help. The best thing that you can do is to take a step back from the situation. Learn to take time for yourself. Find a way to change your lifestyle.

New York psychiatrist Drew M. Slaby, M.D., agrees that stress for a person with diabetes or cardiovascular disease has to be stopped, reduced, and eliminated. He says that the secret to coping with stress is to make stress work for you.

Dr. Slaby's theory is that any stressor can be turned to advantage. In his book, *Sixty Ways to Make Stress Work for You*, Dr. Slaby offers the following nine steps for mastering stress:

1. Get organized. Daily chaos, such as missed appointments and the can't-find-it syndrome, is easy to change. Use an organizer, make lists, and don't let yourself get overextended.

2. Turn a crisis into an opportunity. In every seeming disaster, there is a lesson. If you survive a heart attack, for example, you have the opportunity to change your diet and begin to recover. Be mindful of this concept when the daily disasters strike.

3. Seek a more relaxing environment. Feng Shui has been a hot decorating and environmental design fad based on the belief that by combining the right elements in a space, you restore balance to your life. It's a great idea. By reducing the stress in your home through attractive artwork or comfortable furniture, for example, your personal stress will be eased.

4. Take control of your life. Identify your goals, determine what actions you can take to achieve them, and get started on them. Avoid allowing yourself to create crises in your life, marriage, and work.

5. Avoid surprises. This doesn't mean that you can't have a good old-fashioned surprise party. This refers to not knowing all the information you need about something and suddenly finding yourself in a major mess. For example, not being able to find your destination, or getting there and finding no parking can make you crazy. Plan ahead; it's one of the best stress reducers.

6. Expect the unexpected. If you have to do something or get somewhere, leave time for the unexpected. You will always be faced with things you didn't foresee, so be prepared and don't be caught short.

7. Don't procrastinate. Stress and procrastination go together. Often, stress is caused by anticipation of something that causes you the stress. Step up, deal with the problem, and move on.

8. Let it go. If you dwell on the past, keep in mind that there is nothing you can do about it. The old cliché that "today is the first day of the rest of your life" is pretty accurate.

9. Enlist friends to your side. You need friends to help you recover, and they can also be a great help in reducing your stress. They support you, and they are there for you when you are depressed, or in a quandary. You need great friends. Choose the ones who will be there for you, not those who add to your stress.

In addition, Dr. Slaby recommends the following tips:

- Take note of your stressors, and give some thought to what you might do to help avoid them.
- Realize that you may not be able to change everything or everyone.
- Learn to relax.
- Exercise stress away.
- Don't rush.
- Get enough sleep.
- Avoid negativity.
- Don't obsess about health issues; call your doctor.
- Keep a journal.
- Maintain a healthy diet.
- Live a healthier lifestyle and get your body strong.
- Get psychological therapy if you need it.

REACH OUT FOR HELP

How much of a roadblock is your stress level? If it's normally very high, you might benefit from a formal stress relief program. The decision to join a program is personal, but be sure to talk it over with your doctor and ask if he or she can recommend an appropriate program for you.

stress: a worldwide phenomenon

A recent Roper STARCH worldwide survey of 30,000 people between the ages of thirteen and sixty-five in thirty countries discovered the following:

- Women who work full-time and who have children under the age of thirteen report the greatest stress.
- Nearly one in four mothers who work full-time and who have children under thirteen feel stress almost every day.
- Almost a quarter, 23 percent, of women executives and professionals and 19 percent of their male peers feel "super-stressed."

What if you're not a joiner? Stress and anger management programs teach muscle relaxation, visualization, and breathing exercises, and you can learn these techniques through books or by going online. One excellent website is www.intelihealth.com, which offers complete descriptions of programs and instructions.

Whether you attend a formal program or undertake stress management on your own, the success of any stress management program is related to how much you perceive your need for one.

Help! I Need Somebody. If this sounds like you, many people are uncomfortable with the idea of discussing intimate fears or issues with a stranger, but if you can't manage your stress on your own, ask your doctor to recommend a professional counselor. A psychiatrist may prescribe medication and discuss deeper issues that you may have. Similarly, a psychologist can help you to change behavior and get family counseling, if necessary. A social worker can be a helpful in dealing with practical problems and day-to-day family issues. You might feel more comfortable sitting down with a trusted member of the clergy, who routinely comfort people and guide them through crises.

In *Sixty Ways to Make Stress Work for You*, Dr. Slaby offers this final message: "Making stress work for you won't be achieved only by following sixty ways, seventy ways, or even one thousand ways. Turning the natural stresses of life to your advantage involves combining awareness of physical health, nutrition, exercise, your home or workplace environment, and interpersonal relationships into a plan of your own for stress reduction. After a while, you will develop your own style, techniques, and tricks that will become a pattern for a new and rewarding lifestyle."

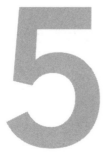

Smoking, Diabetes, and Weight Loss

You face so many roadblocks to weight loss and regaining health as a diabetic that you may need to set priorities to deal with them. Smoking is one roadblock that will take extra effort to overcome. But once you understand how extra-deadly it is for a diabetic, and how much it diminishes your capability to follow the Five-Step Plan, it should (actually it *must*) rise to the top of your list of priorities.

In the past, you might have been all too happy to buy into the myth that stopping will cause weight gain. You can rationalize smoking for any reason, but smoking is far more dangerous than just about any other "everyday" habit you can have. Smoking triples your risk of diabetes, and it diminishes the effect of insulin. It also increases the likelihood of neuropathy, kidney disease, cardiovascular damage, and vision loss. And not everyone gains weight when they quit.

Education is Step One of our Five-Step Plan, so let's start with that—some information that everyone should understand before they light up another cigarette. None of this may come as a surprise to you. Still, the more you hear it, the more likely you are to stop, according to numerous studies.

UNDERSTAND THE SMOKING-DIABETES LINK

Carole Willi, M.D., of the University of Lausanne, Switzerland, and colleagues conducted a systematic review and analysis of studies describing the association between smoking and the incidence of diabetes or other glucose metabolism irregularities that covered thirty years. The data was published in the *Journal of the American Medical Association's December 12, 2007 issue*.

The data indicated that active smokers have a 44 percent increased risk of developing type 2 diabetes compared with nonsmokers. The more you smoke, the greater the risk. People who smoked twenty or more cigarettes a day had a 61 percent increased risk, compared with lighter smokers, who had a 29 percent increased risk.

Death, regular or menthol: Most people associate smoking with cancer. However, its effect on the cardiovascular system and diabetes is stealthy, and your entire organ system can be damaged before you become aware of the extent of the damage. Smoking is an insidious killer. It takes years but by then it is too late.

According to the American Heart Association, more than 440,000 people die each year from smoking-related diseases, and 135,000 additional deaths are linked to the effects of cigarettes on the cardiovascular system. Smokers are two to three times more likely to die of cardiovascular disease than are nonsmokers, according to the American Heart Association.

According to the American Diabetes Association report *Smoking and Diabetes*, cigarette smoking accounts for one out of every five deaths in the United States and is the most important modifiable cause of premature death. Other studies consistently find heightened risk of morbidity and premature death associated with the development of macrovascular complications among smokers. Smoking is also related to the premature development of microvascular complications of diabetes.

The cardiovascular burden of diabetes, especially in combination with smoking, has not been effectively communicated to people with diabetes or to health-care providers, and there is little evidence that this risk factor was being talked about consistently." According to researchers at the Cleveland Clinic Heart Center, "There is no safe amount of smoking. Smokers continue to increase their risk of heart attack the longer they smoke. People who smoke a pack of cigarettes a day have more than twice the risk of heart attack than nonsmokers."

According to the National Institute of Drug Abuse, within 24 hours of quitting, blood pressure and chances of a heart attack decrease. A 35-year-old man who quits smoking will, on average, increase his life expectancy by 5.1 years. The more you smoke, the more likely you are to become atherosclerotic, which results in blocked arteries and reduced blood flow to the heart. If you are diabetic, your diet is poor, and you don't exercise regularly, every cigarette multiplies your risk of developing angina and coronary artery disease.

The peripheral arteries that carry blood to the arms and legs are at increased risk for blockages in smokers, and smoker may suffer symptoms of intermittent claudication (leg pain and cramping due to impaired blood flow). There is also a greater chance of central artery blockages, increasing your risk of stroke.

In addition to increasing your risk of cancer of the lung, mouth, esophagus, and bladder, smoking raises your likelihood of developing chronic obstructive pulmonary disease, emphysema, and gastrointestinal problems, such as gastroesophogeal reflux disease (GERD) and ulcers.

Here are a few more effects of smoking:

- Smoking causes your blood sugar to rise.
- Cholesterol levels and other lipid levels rise as well.
- Smoking can cause high blood pressure.
- Blood vessels are restricted, which can lead to foot ulcers and leg and foot infections in people with diabetes.
- It increases the chance of thrombosis (blood clots).
- Neuropathy (nerve damage) develops or worsens, leading to sexual dysfunction and kidney damage.
- Your immune system becomes compromised, making you more susceptible to infections, colds, bronchitis, and pneumonia.
- It reduces levels of vitamin C in the body, which help your body develop antioxidants (preventing heart disease and cancer), collagen for stronger bones and cells, and healthier gums and also speeds healing of scrapes and burns.
- You inhale 400 different toxins in the smoke and 43 known carcinogens (i.e., cancer-causing agents) every time you take a drag. These include a tar similar to road surfacing tar, the poisonous gas carbon monoxide, arsenic, formaldehyde, ammonia, and many other poisonous compounds. These chemicals circulate in your body, continually putting you at long-term risk, as myriad scientific studies have proven.

- Women who smoke and use oral contraceptives are at higher risk of coronary and peripheral artery diseases, heart attack, and stroke than are nonsmoking women who use oral contraceptives.
- The likelihood of developing complications from medications increases.

All of this increases your chances of dying before your time and makes weight loss more difficult.

UNDERSTAND THE SMOKING–WEIGHT LOSS CONNECTION

If you are a smoker and have diabetes, losing weight will certainly be harder for very specific reasons compared with nonsmoking people with diabetes. Here's why:

- Smokers in general do not have healthy lifestyles—a key to weight loss—so your chances of keeping to the Five-Step Plan are greatly reduced.
- Smoking is directly associated with unhealthy behavior such as lack of (or inability to) exercise.
- Usually, a smoker's diet is low in fruits and vegetables and high in alcohol intake.
- Smokers tend to have more stress in their lives, which often leads to binge eating of fatty and starchy junk foods.

In short, smoking makes it harder to control your weight. But most important of all, smoking greatly increases the chances of fatal complications—sooner.

REVEAL THE SEDUCTIVENESS OF SMOKING

Smoking makes no sense, and even smokers in candid moments will agree. So why do people continue to smoke, knowing what we know about its effects on health?

The short answer is that the active ingredient in tobacco, nicotine, is one of the most addictive compounds yet discovered. According to the National Institute on Drug Abuse (NIDA), a division of the National Institutes of Health, nicotine's effect is caused in part by the drug's stimulation of the adrenal glands and resulting discharge of epinephrine (adrenaline).

the costs of smoking

Smoking has a terrible impact on the economy as well as our medical system. In spite of warnings on cigarette packs, education programs, and disease and death caused by smoking, smokers in the United States alone spend more than $4 billion per year on cigarettes.

Think of the cost of a pack of cigarettes today: about $10 per pack. Rather than striking a match to all of that money, at the end of a week, if you smoke one pack per day and you quit, you'd have at least $70 more to spend on food and entertainment. In one month, you'd save $280; over a year, $3,360! If you smoke more than a pack a day, you do the math.

Despite all the evidence in favor of quitting, 20 percent of Americans still smoke! Despite smoking bans in restaurants, virtually all business, and government offices, you still see people huddle in the cold, on a "break," smoking.

The rush of adrenaline stimulates the body and causes a sudden release of glucose, as well as an increase in blood pressure, respiration, and heart rate, according to the NIDA. Nicotine also suppresses insulin output from the pancreas, which means that smokers are always slightly hyperglycemic; in other words, they have elevated blood sugar levels. The calming effect of nicotine reported by many users is usually associated with a decline in withdrawal effects, rather than the direct effects of nicotine.

Nicotine is what the smoker seeks, because it provokes the release of naturally occurring substances in the brain, such as dopamine, that affect pleasure and pain. Dopamine makes you feel good, and when you stop smoking, you feel miserable, which the body interprets as withdrawal pains.

It may be hard for you to stop smoking for another, more insidious reason. A study released by the Harvard University School of Public Health in January 2007 confirmed a similar study by the Massachusetts Department of Public Health that found that nicotine levels in cigarettes had increased by 11 percent between 1997 and 2005.

"Cigarettes are finely tuned drug delivery devices, designed to perpetuate a tobacco pandemic," Howard Koh, M.D., M.P.H, associate dean for public health practice at Harvard told the Associated Press.

Understanding Physical Addiction

Addiction is a widely misunderstood roadblock to quitting smoking. Addiction to smoking is not caused by an addictive personality. It's caused by nicotine, the active drug in tobacco. A physical addiction is caused by the body's exposure to something that makes it feel good. However, when you take a second dose, the effect is not quite as strong, so you need to increase the dose to equal the effect of the first dose. Over time, you need more and more just to feel normal.

Once your body has decided it likes what you are putting into it—and this can also apply to things like chocolate or coffee—you develop a specific need that makes it hard to turn down another dose. That is called dependency. In the case of smoking, the nicotine makes you feel good, calm, and alert, and your body wants more of the nicotine and can handle whatever you give it. That's building tolerance.

Finally, addiction also is characterized by the decision to continue smoking or other behavior in spite of knowing that the activity in question causes you harm. For example, drinking and driving makes no sense, but people do it. Do you know anyone with a drinking problem who gets into a car and says, "I'm going out on the highway and cause a ten-car pileup?" Of course not.

Because of the way nicotine works in your brain, it's an almost perfect drug when it comes to keeping people hooked and forcing them to increase their daily dose. Think about all of the costs of smoking again and the power of this drug that makes you give up your money as the price goes up. It's so powerful that not only is relapse common, but it almost always takes more than one effort for most people to stop smoking. Fortunately, the more you try to stop, the better the odds are that you will eventually make it.

Understanding Psychological Addiction

There is a difference between physical and psychological addiction, if you believe in the latter. To some this means you are a weak, damaged person who can't help yourself. Psychological addiction is supposed to be a precursor to physical addiction or an excuse to not stop the destructive behavior. There is some evidence that smokers are also risk-takers who try potentially harmful activities for the "rush" these behaviors produce.

Many addiction specialists believe that all drugs that cause addiction are gateway drugs. This means that one substance leads the person to addiction and eventually to multi-drug use. This means that smoking cigarettes might lead to smoking marijuana or using other drugs. For people with diabetes, it really doesn't matter. It's all bad.

QUIT!

Stopping smoking is one of the hardest health-related challenges around, but the following three methods have been proven effective:

1. Join a smoking cessation program.
2. Use nicotine replacement/medication.
3. Quit "cold turkey."

Here are some other options to try:

START: The Centers for Disease Control and Prevention, the office of the Surgeon General, and the Department of Health and Human Services have developed an excellent smoking cessation program, START, that you can downloaded at https://cissecure.nci.nih.gov/ncipubs/details.asp?pid=37. The letters stand for:

S = Set a quit date.

T = Tell family, friends, and coworkers that you are quitting.

A = Anticipate and plan for the challenges you'll face while quitting.

R = Remove cigarettes and other tobacco products from your home, car, and workplace.

T = Talk to your doctor about getting help to quit.

Other websites: www.surgeongeneral.gov/tobacco and www.smokefree .gov offer excellent, useful information on nicotine addiction, hotlines, and contact information to immediately begin the process of quitting smoking.

Support groups: Support groups work well for some people. You can pick up behavioral modification tips that have worked for others that may fit into your lifestyle, such as making lists that remind you of why you want and need to stop smoking or keeping a journal that helps you record times when you needed a cigarette so badly you broke out into a sweat.

Medications: Many medical treatments that claim to help you stop smoking work by using alternate means of nicotine delivery. In other words, get your "dose" in a safer manner. The most common are nicotine patches, nicotine gum, and nicotine nasal inhalers, which can curb the withdrawal symptoms that occur when you stop smoking. The nicotine they give off provides the nicotine you crave, but does not deliver dozens of deadly chemicals every time you inhale. Originally available by prescription, the gum and patches now are available over the counter. There are also lozenges, potions, and fake cigarettes to help break your oral fixation on cigarettes. Do these work? Yes, for some people, but they are costly, and still do not control the need for nicotine so that you can stop using them.

For many years now there has been a search for a "magic pill" to break the tobacco habit. In the past few decades, the antidepressant bupropion (brand name Zyban) has been found to provide the same effect as the replacement devices do by releasing small amounts of dopamine in the brain. The latest and most controversial of these medications is the highly promoted varenicline (brand name Chantix), which became available in 2006. It releases dopamine in the brain, but it is also supposed to block the sites (receptors) in your brain where nicotine activates those positive feelings, which cuts the craving for a cigarette. Chantix is expensive, but it certainly costs less than cigarettes although it is unclear how well it works. In addition, numerous side effects, mostly gastric, have been reported.

The Mayo Clinic's opinion of Chantix is straightforward: For your best chance at quitting smoking with Chantix, you must be committed to your goal. Chantix and other stop-smoking aids may increase the likelihood that you'll quit smoking, but they don't make quitting easy. Most smokers try many times to quit. Most try many different medications and strategies, such as counseling, to stop smoking before they finally succeed. Quitting smoking is very difficult and requires planning and persistence, but it can be done.

Talk to your doctor about your many options for quitting smoking, including counseling. Together, you can decide what stop-smoking medication or strategy might be best for you.

Whatever smoking cessation method you try, you can improve your chances of success by participating in some form of counseling.

There is some validity in acupuncture and hypnosis as antismoking measures, but ask your doctor for a referral to a practitioner of these alternative methods so you know you are seeing someone reputable.

One other note: There are a lot of products on the market and programs outside the mainstream. Some people who have gone to these programs swear by them. Don't do this—especially as a diabetic—without your doctor's approval!

Quitting Cold Turkey

Going "cold turkey" is a slang term for quitting smoking suddenly and completely. You have probably met people who have simply stopped smoking and have been successful—for at least a time. It is not an urban myth that cold turkey often doesn't work because you relapse. Remember that you are fighting an addiction and that addiction specialists consider relapse as part of the definition of recovery.

Fighting an addiction is often so difficult that you can be successful at quitting smoking for a period, then start smoking all over again, then quit again. Remember that the day you stop, you begin to recover your health. So the day you stop again, you start recovering again. Be aware of websites filled with "quit cold turkey" devices. They can be traps for people who are desperate to quit smoking.

QUIT SMOKING WITHOUT GAINING WEIGHT

A common excuse for refusing to stop smoking is that it leads to weight gain. This is frequently true—initially. The reality is that not all people pack on pounds when they stop smoking. Of those who do, most only gain 6 to 8 pounds (3 to 5 kg). Only 10 percent of people who quit gain more than 30 pounds (14 kg). So while most smokers weigh about 4 to 10 pounds (2 to 7 kg) less than nonsmokers, weight gain after quitting smoking generally levels off within 6 months.

Most people gain weight after quitting smoking because smoking increases your metabolic rate, which burns more calories. In addition, quitting may be an excuse to fill the void with candy, alcohol, and sugar-filled soft drinks and foods. The reason is simple: Sugar and carbohydrates have a similar effect on the brain's pleasure centers. In fact, all foods have the same effect, and most of the food we eat also provides needed vitamins, calories, and nutrients.

Losing weight after ceasing smoking is not quite the same as simply going on a diet because years of smoking might have damaged your heart and lungs. Adding weight rapidly could do further damage, leading to or worsening diabetes and increasing the stress on your cardiovascular system. You might feel massive cravings as your system withdraws from nicotine. Talk with your doctor before beginning a weight loss plan after quitting smoking. You'll find a great tool to answer many questions about weight control after quitting smoking at www.smokefree.gov/pubs/FFree3.pdf by the H. Lee Moffitt Cancer Center & Research Institute at the University of South Florida.

If you stay on a program of strict diet and exercise, plus take your supplements and prescribed drugs, it will prevent weight gain.

LIVE SMOKE FREE

Unfortunately the stats show that once smokers quit, it's likely that they will resume smoking. Don't let this throw you. Sometimes you can fall "off the wagon" when you smell a cigarette or have only one. Most experts recommend finding something to distract yourself with when you crave a cigarette. Chewing gum or any sort of physical activity can help. Try to stay away from smokers and don't be embarrassed if you feel you need to say "no" to the offer of a cigarette.

As a diabetic, you have unique things to consider after you quit. It's important that you stay in touch with your health-care provider after you quit. Your diabetes control will probably improve. If so, your health-care provider may want to change your insulin dose or diabetes pill schedule. Similarly, if you are being treated for high blood pressure or high cholesterol levels, your condition may improve so much that your health-care provider may want to change your treatment.

Remember, quitting smoking is probably the most important thing you can do for your health and for the health of those around you.

Diabetes, Family, and Weight Loss

As much as we have discussed the need for conscientious effort on your own part in this weight loss program, your family can also play an important role in helping you achieve success. Integrating diet, exercise, and stress management into a weight loss program isn't simple. Your family can be an important resource in overcoming some of the most difficult behavioral roadblocks described in this book. Living with a chronic disease is not easy. You need all the help you can get, starting with the people you love.

Daily care is not the only critical issue. Preventing progression of the disease is equally important. You will need continuous, patient support to help you face certain practical issues, including the following:

- What is your new diet?
- How mobile are you?
- Are you taking an array of medications?
- Do you have more than one medical problem?
- When can you go back to work?
- Do you need care for other problems?

You and your family may also have to deal with emotional problems that can accompany diabetes (or any chronic disease), such as the following:

- Depression
- Intimacy concerns
- Diminished self-esteem
- Anxiety
- Embarrassment (such as over the number of medications, or shots you must take)
- Denial

FACE THE PROBLEMS TOGETHER

So how can your family help? In what aspects of your diabetes management should your family be involved, either with you or on their own? One American Diabetes Association study of couples in which one partner had type 2 diabetes offers some guidance.

Participants discussed a variety of health-care needs and preferences for type 2 diabetes management. Although being in charge of one's own diabetes was the predominant mode, these couples worked toward a guiding principle of teamwork to maintain their diabetes care. Four core themes emerged from the discussions: educate yourself; talk about the disease, work together, and be your own advocate.

These are good recommendations. Of course, since all families are different, you may have to pick and choose how you and your family work together to help you. Family members of different ages, different family structures, and your weight loss goal can create a different dynamic for every family.

START WITH EDUCATION

Diabetes, like heart disease, is a family disease. You may have been at risk because of your DNA, but even if only one member of the family has diabetes, everyone can be affected. The progression of the disease affects and changes your family's life as well as your own. The impact your illness has on your family is far greater than you might think. It's rare that children aren't scared by a parent's illness, or that the spouse or partner is not affected. Once you are diagnosed with diabetes, it is likely that your family and you will have to make changes in many areas, depending on the severity of your condition.

Then, too, sometimes both you and your family will overreact to the news, either taking it too seriously or not seriously enough.

These are all reasons for which it is vital that your family members know all they can about your diabetes.

Even if your family knows you have diabetes, they need to be aware that you are likely to develop other health problems related to your diabetes. The odds are not in your favor unless you are able to control your risks. This is a key reason for having a good family support system.

Unfortunately, many family members do not fully understand the dangers of diabetes to you and to the family's stability. Hospital personnel routinely warn the families of people who undergo heart surgery or chemotherapy to expect emotional swings or certain practical problems during the recovery period. But diabetes, which is often accompanied by an array of other serious disease conditions and health risks, seldom evokes the same concern or support from family and friends, perhaps because so much of the management of diabetes is done by the patient. Unfortunately, much of the damage to the body caused by diabetes is imperceptible until late in the game, unless a major event, such as a heart attack or diabetic coma, shocks everyone to attention.

When your diabetes is diagnosed, your first instincts may not be to tell anyone or to downplay it. Many people repress or don't communicate the full implications of diabetes—the risk of heart disease, amputation of limbs, kidney failure, and pancreatic disease. Your family deserves to know as much as possible about your situation to offer the support, assistance, and care you need to succeed. Diabetes is a chronic disease with potentially serious complications. Your diabetes can be stable and controlled, but you don't recover from it.

Bring everyone together at one time to talk about the disease. Unless you have this sort of talk, family attitude can be a serious roadblock that has to be overcome for you to be successful in weight loss and enjoy a long life. It's vital that your family understand that diabetes is serious but not a death sentence. While not everyone needs to know all the details (such as sexual dysfunction or diarrhea from your medications), they need to thoroughly understand the basics of how diabetes affects your body. Don't refer them to books or Internet sites or pass out handouts—explain it all to them in your own words. Being informed can dispel any unrealistic concerns anyone may have and will help everyone understand your medication and insulin routines.

After you have educated your family members, make sure that they all really understand what you have said. They may have fears they didn't want to admit, or questions they didn't want to ask. When a family member has a serious diagnosis, either fear or denial can kick in—especially among children. Try to ease their fears or address their denial.

BECOME A RECRUITING OFFICER FOR YOUR CAUSE

Once you have ensured that the family is informed and as comfortable as they can be with the situation—while probably still concerned about you—it's time to become your own best advocate.

Like anyone forming a team or a business organization, someone in your household has to lead the program to manage your diabetes, and it's not going to be your doctor or nutritionist. While they are top-notch consultants, you are the boss and your family now works for you on the "Great Diabetes Control and Weight Loss" project.

While some aspects of your diabetes management program are up to you and your physician, there are a number of ways you can enlist your family's involvement in gaining and maintaining control of your diabetes. Here are some guidelines.

Be fair. Everyone had a different life before and after your diabetes was identified. You can't make the people around you change simply because you have to change. However, you can be aware of their feelings and share yours.

Make assignments. You can "outsource" numerous things to the family to involve them with your diabetes and to reduce their fears. For example, if you need help to go to the store, ask one family member or friend to drive you there. Another person can help you to organize your pills and remind you to take them on time. Another can be your support when you need to talk to someone in the middle of the night. Others can exercise with you, help in meal preparation, and so on. Some family members will be more helpful than others.

Don't "live sick." Unless you are bedridden or actually in the hospital, there is no reason not to try to lead a normal life. Your family members will respond to how you behave, so stay active and stimulated with games, trips to museums, mini-vacations, volunteering, or joining an activity group. You may be dealing with changes in your life, but your overall goal is to lose weight and maintain control of your blood sugars.

Don't refuse to be helped. Few people who have been diagnosed with a chronic illness or who have been released from a hospital want to be hovered over. So often we refuse the help. It's not unusual for family, after you've refused their offers of help, to ask, "If you're so independent and able to take care of yourself, how did you end up in the hospital/so sick?"

To your family, this may seem like a fair question. It really isn't. The point is that accepting their help is an opportunity, not a sign of weakness. You will need to adjust and change each day. Ask for help and accept it graciously when it is offered. You and your support staff have to reach accommodation, and this is an ongoing opportunity to help them understand your need to make lifestyle alterations so they can help you make these life-saving changes.

SOLICIT HELP WITH HEALTHIER EATING

This is one of the key areas your family needs to understand. Your attempts to lose weight can be misinterpreted as "being on a diet" by family members, or they may be resentful of the inconvenience to them or the expense of changes to your diet. Will your new diet change how they eat? Does this mean you can't make pasta or fried foods anymore? These are issues that you have to resolve because you need the help and support of your family to make and maintain essential lifestyle changes.

Do not treat your dietary and lifestyle changes as a recovery plan. Think of it as a permanent lifestyle change for the entire family. Enlisting everyone in your effort to improve your eating habits is important. Teach them about the role of food in maintaining your health and make it positive and goal-oriented. You might consider bringing in your nutritionist to help.

It may not be possible for everyone in the family to share your diet. Children of different ages need certain foods for healthy development, and because they are often very active, they burn more calories than you do. Some members of your family may already have healthy eating and exercise habits. Denying them certain foods that aren't on your approved list is unfair. Finally, if ethnic foods are the norm in your house, you might not be able to share them. Your task is to understand your family's needs and to work out a compromise with them.

dinner out

My coauthor, Larry, remembers his son's reaction when they went out to dinner a year after his heart surgery. After reading each dish on the menu, the son either asked, "Are you allowed to have that?" or declared, "You can't eat that." When they finally came to a mutually acceptable choice, it was clear that his son had paid attention to his father's new dietary needs and was concerned. Most family members will more likely be concerned than bothered by the need for changes in your diet.

This doesn't have to mean separate meals for you and them. You can modify recipes to accommodate everyone. For example, you can all enjoy spaghetti and meatballs together: You can have a small portion of whole-wheat pasta that everyone can eat, a few meatballs, and a green salad or a vegetable on the side, and skip the dessert. This way no one is denied and everyone feels good about helping you. Also consider introducing a new, healthy vegetable or a good source of protein into your meals on a regular basis.

Keep in mind that your culinary modifications, even extensive ones, do not have to make meals a battleground. Explain to your family that much of what you are doing is designed to help you lose weight and overcome roadblocks. Encourage your family to come up with ideas and to participate in the food preparation.

ASK FOR HELP WITH GETTING AROUND

If you are just coming out of the hospital, you may be exhausted or weak. If you have gained weight, you may have been ordered to exercise. Generally, the rule is to resume activity slowly. You need to get up and about and to rebuild your cardiovascular fitness, beginning with light exercise. Family members have a tendency to walk on eggshells, but if you get them to join you in your daily walk or other exercise, they will see your daily improvement, and they will relax and encourage your rehabilitation.

Sometimes, such as after surgery, a diabetic might be restricted from driving or vigorous exercise. For people who are independent, being restricted for even a month can be very frustrating. Family members may be called on to do a lot of transportation duty or perhaps run errands or pick up meds. This may begin to cause friction on both sides. This is often a hidden problem and may become more of a stressor than it should be or pop out when something else is the real problem. Be aware of this and try to plan ahead and set up a schedule that spreads the load around. Also, look for community transportation resources that can help, such as for trips to the market or to doctors.

SOLICIT HELP WITH THE UPS AND DOWNS

It's not unusual for divorced spouses to show up at the hospital or reconnect with a patient because where serious or chronic illness is concerned, the past is less important than human relationships and caring. When life-threatening disease strikes, it's time for all members of the family to put aside past arguments, feuds, and petty problems. Those relatively minor interpersonal issues can often be forgotten when they are seen in the context of something like diabetes. Chronic disease is accompanied by emotional side effects in many cases, and a family support group is a priceless resource for recovery.

Our final message is simple: Don't quit! Don't be afraid to ask for help! Set goals that you can achieve. As you reach each one, your successes and your confidence will build. You can lose weight and regain your health. Don't look back! Your healthy future is only five steps away!

Appendix 1

Side Effects of Common Medications for Diabetes

BIGUANIDES

Side Effects

Stop using metformin and get emergency medical help if you have any of these signs of an allergic reaction: hives; difficulty breathing; or swelling of your face, lips, tongue, or throat. Do not use this drug if you have renal impairment. Additional side effects may include symptoms of lactic acidosis (when the body increases lactic acid too quickly to absorb it), weakness, increasing sleepiness, slow heart rate, feeling of being cold, muscle pain, shortness of breath, stomach pain, feeling light-headed, fainting.

Call your doctor at once if you have any of the following serious side effects:

Feeling short of breath, even with mild exertion; Swelling; Rapid weight gain; Fever; Chills; Body aches; Flu symptoms

Less serious side effects might include the following:

Headache; Muscle pain; Weakness; Mild nausea; Vomiting; Diarrhea; Gas; Stomach pain.

This is not a complete list of side effects; others may occur. Tell your doctor about any unusual or bothersome side effect.

Drug Interactions

You may be more likely to have hyperglycemia (high blood sugar) if you are taking metformin with other drugs that raise blood sugar. Drugs that can raise blood sugar include the following:

Isoniazid (brand name Nydrazid); Diuretics (water pills); Steroids such as prednisone (brand name Deltasone); Phenothiazines such as prochlorperazine (brand name Compazine); Thyroid medicine such as levothyroxine sodium (brand name Synthroid); Birth control pills and other hormones; Seizure medicines such as phenytoin (brand name Dilantin); Diet pills; Medicines to treat asthma, colds, or allergies

You may be more likely to have hypoglycemia (low blood sugar) if you are taking metformin with other drugs that lower blood sugar. Drugs that can lower blood sugar include the following:

Some non-steroidal anti-inflammatory drugs (NSAIDs); Aspirin or other salicylates including Pepto-Bismol; Sulfa drugs such as trimethoprim and sulfamethoxazole (brand name Bactrim); Monoamine oxidase inhibitors (MAOI); Beta-blockers such as atenolol (brand name Tenormin); Probenecid (brand name Benemid)

Some medications may interact with metformin. Tell your doctor if you are taking any of the following drugs:

Furosemide (brand name Lasix); Nifedipine (brand names Adalat, Procardia); Cimetidine (brand name Tagamet); Ranitidine (brand name Zantac); Amiloride (brand name Midamor); Triamterene (brand name Dyrenium); Digoxin (brand name Lanoxin); Morphine (brand names MS-Contin, Kadian); Procainamide (brand names Procan Sr, Pronestyl); Quinidine (brand names Quinidex); Trimethoprim (brand names Bactrim, Septra); Vancomycin (brand name Vancomycin)

This list is not complete, and there may be other drugs that can interact with Metformin. Tell your doctor about all the prescription and over-the-counter medications you use. This includes vitamins, minerals, herbal products, and drugs prescribed by other doctors. Do not start using a new medication without telling your doctor.

Thiazolidinediones (TZDs)

Side Effects
Get emergency medical help if you have any of these signs of an allergic reaction: hives; difficulty breathing; or swelling of your face, lips, tongue, or throat. Stop using pioglitazone (brand name Actos) and call your doctor at once if you have any of the following serious side effects:

Feeling short of breath, even with mild exertion; Swelling or rapid weight gain; Chest pain; General ill feeling; Nausea; Stomach pain; Low fever; Loss of appetite; Dark urine; Clay-colored stools; Jaundice (yellowing of the skin or eyes); Blurred vision; Increased thirst or hunger; Urinating more than usual; Pale skin; Easy bruising or bleeding; Weakness

Continue taking Actos and talk to your doctor if you have any of the following less serious side effects:

Sneezing, runny nose, cough, or other signs of a cold; Headache; Gradual weight gain; Muscle pain; Tooth problems

Side effects other than those listed here may also occur. Talk to your doctor about any side effect that seems unusual or that is especially bothersome.

Drug Interactions
You may be more likely to have hyperglycemia (high blood sugar) if you are taking Actos with the following other drugs that can raise blood sugar:

Isoniazid (brand name Nydrazid); Diuretics (water pills); Steroids such as prednisone (brand name Deltasone); Phenothiazines such as prochlorperazine (brand name Compazine); Thyroid medicine such as levothyroxine sodium (brand name Synthroid); Birth control pills and other hormones; Seizure medicines such as phenytoin (brand name Dilantin); Diet pills; Medicines to treat asthma, colds, or allergies

You may be more likely to have hypoglycemia (low blood sugar) if you are taking Actos with other drugs that lower blood sugar. Drugs that can lower blood sugar include the following:

Some non-steroidal anti-inflammatory drugs (NSAIDs); Aspirin or other salicylates including Pepto-Bismol; Sulfa drugs such as trimethoprim and sulfamethoxazole (brand name Bactrim); Monoamine oxidase inhibitors (MAOI); Beta-blockers such as atenolol (brand name Tenormin); Probenecid (brand name Benemid)

The following drugs can interact with Actos:
Midazolam (brand name Midazolam); Gemfibrozil (brand name Lopid); Rifampin (brand name Rifadin); Furosemide (brand name Lasix); Nifedipine (brand names Adalat, Procardia)

If you are using any of these drugs, you may not be able to use Actos, or you may need dosage adjustments or special tests during treatment.

There may be other medications that can affect Actos. Tell your doctor about all the prescription and over-the-counter medications you use. This includes vitamins, minerals, herbal products, and drugs prescribed by other doctors. Do not start using a new medication without telling your doctor.

DPP-4 INHIBITORS

Side Effects
Get emergency medical help if you have any of these signs of an allergic reaction: hives; difficulty breathing; or swelling of your face, lips, tongue, or throat. Stop using sitagliptin phosphate (brand name Januvia) **and** call your doctor at once if you have fever, sore throat, or headache with severe blistering, peeling, and red skin rash. These could be signs of a serious side effect.

The following less serious side effects may be more likely to occur:
Runny or stuffy nose; Sore throat; Headache; Nausea; Stomach pain; Diarrhea

Side effects other than those listed here also may occur. Talk to your doctor about any side effect that seems unusual or that is especially bothersome.

Drug Interactions

Although data suggest that Januvia is not as likely to cause hypoglycemia (low blood sugar) as some other oral diabetes medications, tell your doctor if you are taking any other drugs that can potentially lower blood sugar, such as the following:

Probenecid (brand name Benemid); Non-steroidal anti-inflammatory drugs (NSAIDs); Aspirin or other salicylates including Pepto-Bismol; Sulfa drugs such as trimethoprim and sulfamethoxazole (brand name Bactrim); Monoamine oxidase inhibitors (MAOI); Beta-blockers such as atenolol (brand name Tenormin)

Before you take Januvia, tell your doctor if you are also taking digoxin (brand name Lanoxin). You may not be able to take Januvia, or you may require a dosage adjustment or special monitoring.

There may be other drugs not listed that can affect Januvia. Tell your doctor about all the prescription and over-the-counter medications you use, including vitamins, minerals, herbal products, and drugs prescribed by other doctors. Do not start using a new medication without telling your doctor.

Januvia comes in tablets; patients take the medication once daily. It has not been studied in children less than eighteen years old, according to the patient information sheet for this drug.

EXENATIDE (BRAND NAME BYETTA)

Side Effects

Get emergency medical help if you have any of these signs of an allergic reaction: hives; difficulty breathing; or swelling of your face, lips, tongue, or throat.

Call your doctor at once if you have severe pain in your upper stomach that spreads to your back, accompanied by nausea, vomiting, and a rapid heart rate. These could be symptoms of pancreatitis.

Less serious side effects may include the following:

Nausea; Vomiting; Heartburn; Diarrhea; Loss of appetite; Weight loss; Dizziness; Headache; Jittery feeling

This is not a complete list of side effects; others may occur. Tell your doctor about any unusual or bothersome side effect.

Know the signs of low blood sugar (hypoglycemia) and how to recognize them. A severe hypoglycemic episode can be fatal. Hypoglycemia can occur if you do not consume sufficient calories. The signs include the following:

Hunger; Headache; Confusion; Irritability; Drowsiness; Weakness; Dizziness; Tremors; Sweating; Fast heartbeat; Seizure (convulsions); Fainting; Coma

Always keep a source of sugar available in case you have symptoms of low blood sugar. These include orange juice, glucose gel, candy, or milk. If you have severe hypoglycemia and cannot eat or drink, use an injection of glucagon. Your doctor can give you a prescription for a glucagon emergency injection kit and tell you how to give the injection. A MedicAlert bracelet is a good idea for some people and you can find out more about them at www.medicalert.com. Let your family and close friends know about these symptoms and keep a list of emergency contacts and your medications in your wallet.

Drug Interactions

Before using Byetta, tell your doctor if you use any oral diabetes medications such as the following. You may need a dose adjustment:

Acetohexamide (brand name Dymelor); Chlorpropamide (brand name Diabinese); Glimepiride (brand name Amaryl); Glipizide (brand name Glucotrol); Glyburide (brand name Diabeta); Tolazamide (brand name Tolinase); Tolbutamide (brand name Orinase)

Your doctor will tell you if any of your medication doses need to be changed.

There may be other drugs that can interact with Byetta. Tell your doctor about all the prescription and over-the-counter medications you use. This includes vitamins, minerals, herbal products, and drugs prescribed by other doctors. Do not start using a new medication without telling your doctor.

SULFONYLUREAS

Side Effects

The use of sulfonylurea antidiabetic agents has been reported, but not proven in all studies, to increase the risk of death from heart and blood vessel disease. Patients with diabetes are already more likely to have these problems if they do not control their blood sugar. Some sulfonylureas, such as glyburide (brand names Micronase, Diabeta) and gliclazide (brand name Diamicron), can have a positive effect on heart and blood vessel disease. It is important to know that problems may occur, but it is also not known if other sulfonylureas, particularly tolbutamide (brand name Orinase), help to cause these problems. It is known that if blood sugar is not controlled, such problems may occur.

Along with their desirable effects, sulfonylureas may cause some unwanted effects. Although not all of these side effects may occur, if they do occur you may need medical attention.

If you experience convulsions (seizures) or lose consciousness, make sure that you or someone else calls your doctor immediately, and that you go to the emergency room as soon as possible.

Check with your doctor as soon as possible if you experience any of the following:

Low blood sugar; Anxiety; Behavior similar to being drunk; Blurred vision; Cold sweats; Confusion; Cool pale skin; Difficulty in concentrating; Drowsiness; Excessive hunger; Fast heartbeat; Headache; Nausea; Nervousness; Nightmares; Restless sleep; Shakiness; Slurred speech; Unusual tiredness or weakness; Unusual weight gain

Peeling of skin and skin redness, itching, or rash are less common side effects that should be brought to your doctor's attention immediately, as should the following rare side effects:

Chest pain; Chills; Coughing up blood; Dark urine; Fever; Fluid-filled skin blisters; General feeling of illness; Increased amounts of phlegm; Increased sweating; Light-colored stools; Pale skin; Sensitivity to the sun; Shortness of breath; Sore throat; Thinning of the skin; Unusual bleeding or bruising; Unusual tiredness or weakness; Yellow eyes or skin

Other side effects may occur that usually do not need medical attention. These side effects may go away during treatment as your body adjusts to the medicine. However, check with your doctor if any of the following side effects continue or are bothersome:

Changes in sense of taste; Constipation; Diarrhea; Dizziness; Increased amount of urine or more frequent urination; Heartburn; Increased or decreased appetite; Passing gas; Stomach pain, fullness, or discomfort; Vomiting; Difficulty in focusing the eyes; Increased sensitivity of skin to sun

Some patients who take chlorpropamide (brand name Diabinese) may retain water. Check with your doctor as soon as possible if any of the following signs occur:

Depression; Swelling or puffiness of face, ankles, or hands

Other side effects not listed above may also occur in some patients. If you notice any other side effects, check with your doctor.

Side Effects Related to Repaglinide (Brand Name Prandin)

Although not all of the following side effects may occur, if they do occur they may need medical attention.

If you experience convulsions (seizures) or lose consciousness, make sure that you or someone else calls your doctor immediately and that you go to the emergency room as soon as possible.

Check with your doctor as soon as possible if any of the following side effects occur:

Cough; Fever; Low blood sugar; Anxious feeling; Behavior change similar to being drunk; Blurred vision; Cold sweats; Confusion; Cool, pale skin; Difficulty in thinking; Drowsiness; Excessive hunger; Fast heartbeat; Headache; Nausea; Nervousness; Nightmares; Restless sleep; Shakiness; Slurred speech; Unusual tiredness or weakness; Pain in the chest; Runny or stuffy nose; Shortness of breath; Sinus congestion with pain; Sneezing; Sore throat; Bloody or cloudy urine; Burning, painful, or difficult urination; Chest pain; Chills; Frequent urge t o urinate; Problems with teeth; Skin rash; Itching; Hives; Tearing of eyes; Tightness in chest; Trouble breathing; Vomiting; Wheezing

If you experience any of the following rare side effects, tell your doctor:

Black, tarry stools; Blood in stools; Fast or irregular heartbeat; Hoarseness; Lower back or side pain; Pinpoint red spots on skin; Unusual bleeding or bruising

Other side effects may occur that usually do not need medical attention. These may go away during treatment as your body adjusts to the medicine; however, check with your doctor if any of the following side effects continue or are bothersome:

Back pain; Diarrhea; Joint pain; Constipation; Feeling of burning on the skin; Numbness; Tightness; Tingling; Warmth on the skin; Indigestion

Other side effects not listed above may also occur in some patients. If you notice any other effects, check with your doctor.

ACARBOSE (BRAND NAME PRECOSE)

Side Effects
Side effects cannot be anticipated because they are often a reaction to a component in a medication that you have never been exposed to before. If they develop or change in intensity, tell your doctor as soon as possible. Only your doctor can determine if it is safe for you to continue taking Precose. Side effects usually are rare, and usually appear during the first few weeks of therapy, after which they gradually become less intense and less frequent over time. The most common side effects are abdominal pain, diarrhea, and gas.

Special Warnings about Precose
Every three months during your first year of treatment, your doctor will take a blood sample to determine how your liver is reacting to Precose. While you are taking Precose, you should check your blood and urine periodically for the presence of abnormal glucose levels.

Even people with well-controlled diabetes may find that stresses such as injury, infection, surgery, or fever can lead to uncontrolled blood sugar. If this happens to you, your doctor may recommend that Precose be discontinued temporarily and injected insulin used instead.

Taken alone, Precose does not cause hypoglycemia (low blood sugar), but when you take it in combination with other medications such as chlorpropamide (brand name Diabinese) or glipizide (brand name Glucotrol), or with insulin, your blood sugar may fall too low. If you have any questions about combining Precose with other medications, be sure to discuss them with your doctor.

If you are taking Precose along with other diabetes medications, be sure to have some source of glucose, such as glucose tablets, available in case you experience symptoms of mild or moderate low blood sugar. Note: Table sugar won't work in this situation because Precose inhibits its absorption. Symptoms of mild hypoglycemia may include a cold sweat, fast heartbeat, fatigue, headache, nausea, and nervousness; more severe hypoglycemia is characterized by coma, pale skin, and shallow breathing.

Severe hypoglycemia is an emergency. Contact your doctor immediately if the symptoms occur.

Drug Interactions
When you take Precose with certain other drugs, the effects of either could be increased, decreased, or altered. It is especially important to check with your doctor before taking Precose with the following:

Airway-opening drugs such as albuterol (brand name Proventil); Calcium-channel blockers (heart and blood pressure medications) such as diltiazem (brand name Cardizem) and nifedipine (brand name Procardia); Charcoal tablets; Digestive enzyme preparations such as pancrelipase (brand name Creon 20) and Donnazyme; Digoxin (brand name Lanoxin); Estrogens (brand name Premarin); Rifampin and isoniazid (brand name Rifamate); Major tranquilizers such as prochlorperazine (brand name Compazine) and thioridazine HCl (brand name Mellaril); Nicotinic acid (brand names Nicobid, Nicolar); Oral contraceptives; Phenytoin (brand name Dilantin); Steroid medications such as prednisone (brand name Deltasone); Thyroid medications such as levothyroxine sodium (brand name Synthroid); Diuretics (water pills) such as methyclothiazide (brand name Enduron)

Special Information if You Are Pregnant or Breastfeeding
The effects of Precose during pregnancy have not been adequately studied. If you are pregnant or plan to become pregnant, tell your doctor immediately. Since studies suggest the importance of maintaining normal blood sugar levels during pregnancy, your doctor may prescribe injected insulin. It is not known whether Precose appears in breast milk. Because many drugs do appear in breast milk, you should not take Precose while breastfeeding.

Appendix 2

Quick Recipes

The following are some good recipes for people with prediabetes or type 2 diabetes. They were provided to us by chef Liz Scott, nationally recognized professional chef and cookbook author. Her down-to-earth approach to healthy eating has won accolades for her published works from the Independent Publisher Book Award in Health, Medicine, and Nutrition, *Foreword* Magazine's Cookbooks of the Year, and the National Health Information Award for Patient Education Information. As the author of *The Sober Kitchen* and *Sober Celebrations*, she was honored by the Johnson Institute in Washington, DC as an innovator of recovery eating and is a coveted speaker at health conventions and conferences. Her forthcoming titles include *The Complete Idiot's Guide to High Fiber Cooking* and the fully illustrated *Zero Proof Cocktails* with Ten Speed Press.

BREAKFAST
Scrambled Egg and Salsa Wrap
Makes 1 serving

1 teaspoon unsalted butter

2 large eggs

1 tablespoon (15 ml) water

Salt and pepper to taste

One 8-inch (20.3 cm) whole wheat wrap, warmed

1 tablespoon (15 g) shredded reduced-fat Cheddar cheese

1 tablespoon (20 g) prepared salsa

1. Melt the butter in a medium frying pan, preferably nonstick.
2. Whisk together the eggs, water, salt, and pepper in a bowl. Pour the egg mixture into the pan all at once, reduce heat to medium-low, and stir with a wooden spoon until thickened, about 1 minute.
3. Spoon eggs into the wrap, sprinkle with the cheese and salsa, and fold over. Serve immediately.

Apple-Cinnamon Oatmeal

Makes 1 serving

½ cup (40 g) old-fashioned or Irish oats

½ medium apple, diced

Dash of ground cinnamon

½ teaspoon unsalted butter

¼ cup (60 ml) soy milk

1. Prepare oats according to package directions, adding the diced apple and cinnamon during the last minute, stirring well.
2. Transfer to a serving bowl, dot with the butter, and pour the soy milk around the edge. Serve immediately.

LUNCH

Almond-Chicken Salad

Makes 1 serving

1 cup (140 g) cooked, diced chicken breast, chilled

½ small celery stalk, diced

8 whole almonds

1 tablespoon (14 g) light mayonnaise

Dash of paprika

Salt and pepper to taste

1. In a mixing bowl, gently combine all ingredients with a rubber spatula. Transfer to a plate lined with lettuce leaves, if desired. Serve with whole grain crackers or rice cakes.

Avocado-Shrimp Surprise

Makes 1 serving

¾ cup (150 g) cooked baby salad shrimp

2 teaspoons (10 g) light mayonnaise

1 teaspoon cocktail sauce

½ avocado, pitted and skin removed

Shredded lettuce

1 scallion, trimmed and thinly sliced

Low-carb whole wheat roll

1. In a small bowl combine the shrimp, mayonnaise, and cocktail sauce.
2. Place the avocado on the lettuce and fill with the shrimp salad. Sprinkle with the scallions and serve with the roll.

Tuna and White Bean Salad

Makes 1 serving

One 3-ounce (85 g) can solid white tuna in spring water, drained

⅔ cup (170 g) canned cannelini beans, rinsed and drained

Freshly ground black pepper

Extra virgin olive oil for drizzling

1 tablespoon (4 g) chopped fresh parsley

1 plum tomato, thinly sliced

1. In a small bowl gently combine the tuna, beans, and pepper, and transfer to the middle of a serving plate.
2. Drizzle with the olive oil, sprinkle the parsley over, and place the tomato slices around. Serve immediately.

DINNER ENTREES

Best Ever Turkey Burger

Makes 1 serving

4 ounces (114 g) lean ground turkey

2 tablespoons (7.5 g) cooked chopped spinach, well drained

1 egg white

2 white mushrooms, roughly chopped

1 teaspoon dried cranberries, roughly chopped

Pinch of dried rubbed sage

Salt and pepper to taste

1. In a small mixing bowl, stir together all the ingredients until well combined. Form into a burger-size patty and refrigerate for 20 minutes.
2. Grill or broil turkey burger until well browned and no longer pink inside, about 3 minutes per side. Serve with Oven Fried Sweet Potatoes (page 216).

Lemon and Herb Baked Flounder

Makes 1 serving

1 medium flounder or sole fillet

1 teaspoon lemon juice

½ teaspoon olive oil

Pinch of dried thyme

Salt and pepper to taste

1. Preheat the oven to 400°F (200°C, or gas mark 6). Line a baking pan with foil and coat lightly with cooking spray.
2. Place the fillet flat in middle of pan. Sprinkle with the lemon juice, oil, thyme, salt, and pepper. Bake until firm to the touch, about 12 minutes. Serve immediately.

Peppered Steak with Garlic Sauce

Makes 1 serving

1 filet mignon beef steak

3 teaspoons crushed black peppercorns

Salt to taste

1 teaspoon olive oil

1 garlic clove, minced

1 teaspoon red wine vinegar

2 tablespoons (28 ml) red wine grape juice

1. Coat the steak on both sides with the crushed pepper and season to taste with salt.
2. Heat a heavy skillet over high heat and add the olive oil. Add the steak and cook over high heat to brown, about 2 minutes per side. Cover and reduce the heat to medium-low. Continue cooking until desired doneness is reached,

3 to 4 more minutes for medium-rare. Transfer the steak to a serving plate and return the skillet to the heat.

3. Add the garlic and cook over medium heat for 1 minute. Add the vinegar and grape juice, stirring and scraping the pan as the sauce simmers for another minute. Pour the sauce over the steak and serve.

SIDE DISHES

Oven Fried Sweet Potatoes

Makes 1 serving
One 3.5-ounce (100 g) sweet potato
Dash ground cinnamon
Salt and pepper to taste

1. Preheat the oven to 375°F (190°C, or gas mark 5). Lightly coat a baking pan with cooking spray.
2. Peel the sweet potato and remove the ends. Cut into ¼-inch (6 mm) circles and place on the baking pan in a single layer. Sprinkle with the cinnamon, salt, and pepper, and bake until tender and golden around the edges, about 30 minutes, turning the potato slices over halfway through.
3. Drain on a paper towel and serve immediately.

Crumb-Topped Broccoli Bake

Makes 1 serving
1 cup (71 g) frozen or fresh broccoli florets, cooked
Salt and pepper to taste
1 tablespoon (15 ml) light sour cream
1 teaspoon melted butter
1½ tablespoons (10 g) bread crumbs

1. Place the broccoli in a small flame-proof baking dish. Sprinkle with the salt and pepper and dot with the sour cream. Combine the melted butter and bread crumbs, and sprinkle over the top.
2. Place under an oven broiler set to low, and cook until heated through and golden on top, 4 to 5 minutes. Serve immediately.

About the Authors

Frederic J. Vagnini M.D., FACS

Dr. Fred Vagnini is unique among modern medical practitioners. He is a board-certified cardiovascular surgeon whose understanding of the ravages of cardio-vascular diseases is grounded in twenty years as a cardiac surgeon. Today his practice is dedicated to preventing these diseases through nutrition, lifestyle counseling, and health education. His popular call-in show, *The Heart Show*, on WOR-710 (NY) every Sunday is a mix of sound health maintenance advice and humor that has attracted regular listeners is the tens of thousands.

Dr. Vagnini's commitment to health education is further evidenced by his several published books: *The Carbohydrate Addict's Healthy Heart Program*, a *New York Times* bestseller, and *Count Down Your Age*, which takes the advances of modern medical science and common sense and lays out a plan for personal longevity. His most recent book gets its title from the sign-off slogan he has used on his radio show for twenty years: *Your Health Is in Your Own Hands.*

Dr. Vagnini's other books are:
Yes! You Can Stop Heart Disease before It Starts

Understanding Insulin Resistance
30 Minutes a Day to a Healthy Heart
The Side Effects Bible
Overcoming Metabolic Syndrome

"Dr. V," as he is familiarly called by friends and clients, received his medical degree from St. Louis University Medical School, St Louis, followed by specialty training at Downstate and Columbia Presbyterian Medical Centers, New York. He also served in the U.S. Army at the rank of Lieutenant Colonel. He is an assistant professor of surgery at Long Island Jewish/North Shore University Medical Center on Long Island.

Dr. Vagnini may be reached any day of the week, either in his Park Avenue office in Manhattan or his Westbury Long Island office, where he is the Medical Director of the Heart, Diabetes and Weight Loss Centers of New York. Call 1-888-HEART-90 or visit his websites: www.vagnini.com and www.drvblog.com.

Lawrence D. Chilnick

Mr. Chilnick is a publishing executive, editor, author, teacher, journalist, broadcaster, and author of popular cookbooks, business and health reference books, electronic products, audiotapes, and videos. Print and electronic products he has created and authored, such as the 17 million copy *New York Times bestseller*, *The Pill Book* (Bantam), have become standard reference works that are still in print after more than two decades.

His latest book, *The First Year: Heart Disease* (Da Capo) for people who have recently been diagnosed with cardiovascular disease, was published in February 2008.

Mr. Chilnick often consults to start-up publishing companies and is currently developing a new line of children's books for VanitaBooks in Akron, Ohio. From 2004 through 2006, he was editorial director of Cleveland Clinic Press, responsible for development of more than twenty-five books.

Mr. Chilnick has published or collaborated with many of the leading authorities in the fields of cooking, traditional and alternative health care, psychiatry, substance abuse, adolescent and family issues, eating disorders, employee health care, pharmacology, law, business/computer technology management, and library reference. He specializes in the development of new products and has been especially successful in making inefficient corporate publishing operations more profitable.

In addition, from 1997 through 2003, Mr. Chilnick taught introductory and advanced graduate school level publishing courses and writing workshops in a variety of settings. As adjunct professor at the New York University School of Continuing and Professional Education, he taught the Capstone/Thesis Course for Master in Publishing candidates, Book Packaging and the Role of The Independent Press. The courses there resulted in the publication of several trade books, including the award-winning bestsellers *Looneyspoons* and *The Sober Kitchen Cookbooks*, and *The Good News About Depression.*

Major executive positions held include publisher of Thomson Publishing's Auerbach Information Technology Management products, vice president and publisher at Reed-Elsevier. Mr. Chilnick directed book buying and new book business development operations at QVC and founded the PIA Press, which developed imprints at Random House, Berkeley, and Bantam.

Acknowledgments

There are many people in my life that are important to me and my work. First of all with regard to this publication, which I am extremely proud of, I would like to thank Colleen O'Shea, my agent who has been a strong force in helping myself and my co-author get through this process. The editors at Fair Winds Press, especially Jill Alexander, have been extremely helpful and have been committed to making this a successful project. My co-author and writer, Lawrence Chilnick, has been the backbone of this piece of work, which I consider one of the significant things I have accomplished in my medical career. Larry has been able to capture my work, my words, and put it into print where it is easily understandable and hopefully helpful to the hundreds of thousands of people out there with prediabetes and diabetes.

A sincere and special note of thanks to Maria Santoro and Giuliana Mazzeo, my medical nutritionists and diabetes educators. They have successfully managed several thousand of my patients. In addition, they both have contributed significantly to this book. Their work is outlined in the food and menu sections, and is of major importance.

Dr. Rachel and Richard Heller, friends and colleagues, started me into the publishing aspect of medicine by allowing me to co-author the best-selling book, *The Carbohydrate Addict's Healthy Heart*. The Heller's have been way ahead of their time talking about the importance of insulin as it relates to diet, weight loss, and cardiovascular disease. I am eternally grateful for their friendship, knowledge and advice.

My family, sisters Ann and Grace; and daughters, Grace and Clare, have been instrumental and a force behind my commitment to my work and patients.

My nephew, Dan Cajigas, has not only been a loyal friend and nephew, but he has been CEO and CFO of my centers, vitamin companies, and co-host of my radio shows. He has managed to pull everything together with a 24-7 commitment that has made the centers improve and has allowed me to dedicate myself to helping the millions of people through the media and my Centers to be healthy and hopefully to live a longer life.

Dr. Mary Infantino, director of my Women's Health Initiative has been a force in allowing my centers to excel and go beyond my capabilities. Mary is a professor and program director at CW Post University of the Nurse Practitioning Program, and she has brought to me a teaching program with an outstanding number of students. Her colleague, also working at my center, is Waitline D. Deroux-Smith, who has been outstanding in the management of my patients. Dr. Mary has brought to me a number of talented students who have helped me in managing my patients. Particularly outstanding in the student area is my now-colleague, Susan Laforte, who is not only an outstanding student, but has become a brilliant clinician and has shown the compassion and commitment to be a force in the medical profession. It is through these young ladies as well as through my broadcasting and writings that I believe I will have a significant legacy. My teachings in all of these areas, especially in the area of the nurse practitioners with Mary, Waitline, and Susan, hopefully will last for many, many years.

My writer, Goeffrey Proud, as the editor of my monthly newsletter, *Dr. V's Longevity Report*, has worked with me over the last twenty years and was co-editor and writer of my book, *Your Health is in Your Own Hands*.

I would like to thank the WOR Radio Company, especially Bob and Jen Buckley and Jerry Crowley, for allowing me to broadcast on this radio station for over twenty years. This has been an important part of my health education program. Finally, I would like to thank the thousands of patients seen at my centers who are giving me the privilege of giving them my new concept of medical care and all of the employees at my centers, who have given beyond the expected. Especially Paulette Sonds and Mildred Nappo.

Fredric J. Vagnini, MD, FACS

I would also would also like to thank the following people for their continual assistance, professional expertise, and support during the writing and editing of this book. First and foremost are the two nutritionists Maria Santoro and Giuliana Mazzeo who helped develop our dietary program, returned calls and e-mails quickly and checked and rechecked. Additional thanks to Chef Liz Scott who provided the original recipes featured in the books. And also to three friends/editors; Patricia Fernberg, Carol Cartaino and Jennifer Bright Reich, whose skills are superb and enhanced the voice of this book with careful reading and feedback.

I too, am also especially grateful for the skill, support and especially the patience of our agent, Coleen O'Shea. More than once she kept us on track and focused. No matter what happens, she can fix it.

I also wish to especially thank my cardiology and other medical sources including Michael Lux, M.D. Curtis M. Rimmerman, M.D. Richard Cohen, M.D. Harold Solomon, M.D., Andrew Slaby, M.D. They have all been great teachers and healers.

Finally but not last, working on this book with "Dr. V" has been a grand experience combining education, with his understanding and voluminous knowledge base that made working on this book an exceptional experience.

Lawrence D. Chilnick

Resources

Diabetes Prevention: Diet and Weight Loss Centers
Personal website of Dr. Frederic J. Vagnini and Daniel L. Cajigas
www.vagnini.com

Dr. V's Blog
The blog, podcast, and webcast of Dr. Frederic J. Vagnini
www.drvblog.com

The Beating Diabetes Twitter Account
Updates from Dr. Frederic J. Vagnini on information pertaining to the book
www.twitter.com/beatingdiabetes

Energy Transformations
Website of Aleta St. James, energy healer and author of *Life Shift, Let Go and Live Your Dreams*
www.aletastjames.com

N3 Oceanic
Makers of the Res-Q brand products
www.n3inc.com

Willner Chemists
Makers and pharmaceutical representatives of nutritional supplements
www.willner.com

Kyolic Aged Garlic Extract
Part of Wakunaga Nutritional Supplements
www.kyolic.com

Orosine
A product of the Res-Q natural supplement line of products
www.orosine.com

WOR News Talk Radio
Discussions of news, food, health, travel, the economy, and more
www.wor710.com

The American Diabetes Association
www.diabetes.org

T. A. Sciences
Cell rejuvenation through telomerase activation (T.A.)
www.tasciences.com

The Greta Blackburn Fit Camp and Ms. Fitness Fan Club
Website of Greta Blackburn, founding editor of *Ms. Fitness Magazine* and founder/director of FITCAMPS – "training symposiums for fitness professionals." She is also the executive vice president of business development for T.A. Sciences.
www.gretablackburn.com

The American Heart Association

www.americanheart.org

The Carbohydrate Addict's Official Home Page

Website devoted to offering advice towards managing carbohydrate intake

www.carbohydrateaddicts.com

Bioenergy Life Science, Inc.

Makers and producers of ribose-based supplements

www.bioenergy.com

Enzymatic Therapy, Inc.

Makers and producers of enzymatic therapy supplements

www.enzymatictherapy.com

www.enzy.com

alpha betic

Makers and producers of nutritional supplements for people with diabetes

www.alphabetic.com

Index

C

calories, counting of, 93, 159
candidasis, 27
    blood test for, 53
    nutrition and, 115, 120
capillary filling, testing of, 57
carbo-drifting, 27, 159
carbohydrates
    carbohydrate addiction, 27
    endorphins and, 93–94
    glucose and, 36
    in lifestyle self-assessment test,
        144
    nutrition and, 90–91, 92, 97–98
    phaseolamin and, 114
    in specific foods, 106
cardiac exercise tolerance test, 56
cardio metabolic risk, 31
cardio-CRP, 41
cardiovascular health
    complications of, 28–29
    exercise and, 130
    lifestyle changes and, 151
    link with diabetes, 32–33, 36–39
    nutraceuticals for, 119–120
    providing doctor with history of,
        47–48
    smoking and, 186–188
    women and, 167–173
carotid duplex, 57
central nervous system, information
    for doctor, 49

cerebrovascular disease, in women,
    174
Chalmers, Dr. Karen, 166–167
Chantix, 192
children, metabolic syndrome and, 40
Chilnick, Lawrence, 131, 133
cholesterol, 91
    healthy levels of, 51
    women and, 169, 175
chromium, 114
cigarettes. *See* smoking
circuit training, 128, 130
co-enzyme Q10, 116
colesevelam hydrochloride, 65
continuous subcutaneous insulin
    infusion therapy, 154
coronary calcium scoring, 57
coronary computer-assisted
    tomographic (CAT) scan, 56–57
coronary microvascular syndrome,
    171
C-reactive protein (CRP), 41
crisis, turning into opportunity, 182
cross training, 128
cyanosis, testing for, 57

D

dance aerobics, 128
Dansinger, Dr. Michael L., 168
death, risk of, 30
Defronzo, Dr. Ralph A., 70

tips for stocking pantry, 106–109
"Guidelines for Preventing
    Cardiovascular Disease in Women"
    (AHA), 172–173

H

h2 blockers, 27
health clubs, 136–137
health issues, informing doctor about,
    49–50
Heart, Diabetes and Weight Loss
    Center of New York, 24
heart disease. See cardiovascular
    disease
Heart Outcomes Prevention Evaluation
    (HOPE) study, 66
heavy metals
    blood tests for levels of, 53
    toxicity and, 28
Heidelberg test, 86
Helicobacter pylori, 53
hemoglobin A1C
    meaning of test results, 54–55
    nutrition and, 84, 97–98
herbs and spices, recommended, 107
high blood pressure. See hypertension
high-sensitivity C-reactive protein
    (CRP), healthy levels of, 51
home blood monitoring, 55–56
homocysteine
    blood tests for, 53

healthy levels of, 51
    nutraceuticals for, 119–120
hormone replacement therapy (HRT),
    169–170
hormones, women and cardiovascular
    disease, 168–170
Humalog, 65, 74
hyperglycemia
    exercise and, 125
    metabolic syndrome and, 25
    postprandial, 26, 40–41
hyperinsulinemia, 26, 40–41
hyperlipidemia, 41
hypertension, 39, 51
    metabolic syndrome and, 25
    nutraceuticals for, 119–120
    women and, 175
hypertriglyceridemic waist, 32
hypnosis, smoking cessation and, 193
hypochlorhydria, 27
hypoglycemia, exercise and, 125
hypothyroidism, 120

I

impaired fasting glucose (IFG), 35
impaired glucose tolerance (IGT), 35
incretin mimetics, 62, 65–66, 69–71
    side effects and drug interactions,
    206–207
infections, slow healing of, 41

inflammation, nutraceuticals for, 119–120

insulin, 34–35

    brand names of, 65, 74

    continuous subcutaneous infusion therapy, 154

    nutraceuticals for, 118–119

    reasons for injecting, 74–75

    weight loss and fluctuating levels of, 25

insulin manipulation, by women, 166–167

insulin pump, 154

insulin resistance, 34–35

insurance issues

    choice of doctor and, 44

    help with medical expenses, 79

    lack of and early morbidity, 174

integrative medicine, 112

intestinal dysbiosis, 27, 120

inversion tables, 135

ischemia, silent, 32–33

J

Janumet, 69

Januvia, 65, 68, 69

    side effects and drug interactions, 205–206

journaling, 138

K

kickboxing, 128

kidney disease, 42

Koh, Dr. Howard, 189

Kyolic (aged garlic), 117

L

lamb, recommended, 108

Lantus, 65, 74

legs

    examination of, 57

    informing doctor about pain in, 49–50

legumes, recommended, 107

Levemir, 74

lifestyle changes, as step five, 139–156

    examples of change, 151–156

    making game plan for, 156

    preparing for, 140–141

    self-assessment test of lifestyle, 143–147

    setting priorities for change, 148–151

    stating readiness to change, 141–142

    stress management and, 182

lipids, 41

    blood tests for, 52

    nutraceuticals for, 119–120

lipotoxicity, 35

pork, recommended, 108

postprandial dysmetabolism, 41

postprandial hyperglycemia, 26, 40–41

postprandial hyperlipidemia, 41

potatoes, recommended, 109

poultry, recommended, 108

pramlintide acetate injection, 65, 75

Prandin, 65, 72

    side effects and drug interactions, 209–210

Precose, 65, 72–73

    side effects and drug interactions, 210–211

prediabetes, 17, 19, 36

    cardiovascular disease and, 38–39

    exercise and, 122

    numbers of people with, 20

pregnancy, Precose and, 211

Premarin, 169–170

priorities, setting for lifestyle change, 148–151

    cardiovascular health, 151

    improved nutrition, 149–150

    motivation, 148–149

    setting goal with doctor, 149

    stop smoking, 150–151

probiotics, 115

procrastination, avoiding, 182

protein wasting, 31

proteins, nutrition and, 91, 92

psychiatrists/psychologists, stress management and, 184

psychological roadblocks, 29, 190–191

R

ramipril, 66

Rated-Perceived Exercise (RPE) Scale, 131

recipes

    breakfast, 212–213

    dinner, 214–216

    lunch, 213–214

    side dishes, 216

recumbent exercise bikes, 134

refrigerator items, list of basic, 107

relaxing environment, stress management and, 182

repaglinide, 65, 72

    side effects and drug interactions, 209–210

resistance exercise, 129, 130

respiratory conditions, information for doctor, 49

resting metabolic rate, measuring of, 85–86

resveratrol, 115–116

retinal examination, 57

rosiglitazone, 65, 68

rowing machine, 130, 135

S

W

waistline. *See* hypertriglyceridemic waist; visceral adipose tissue

walking, as exercise, 127–128

in lifestyle self-assessment test, 143, 145

weekly meal suggestions, 100–101

weight cycling, 18

weight loss

money-saving aspects of, 19–20

therapeutic benefits of, 17

weight management

challenges of, 24–29

nutraceuticals for, 118–119

weight training, 128

Weight Watchers, 137

Welchol, 65

Willi, Dr. Carole, 186

Williams, Dr. Redford, 178

Women's Ischemic Syndrome Evaluation study (WISE), 171

women's issues, 165–175

cardiovascular disease and hormones, 167–170

cardiovascular disease symptoms, 170–172

cardiovascular disease treatments, 172–173

cerebrovascular disease and, 174

diabetic ketoacidosis, 174

ethnic groups and, 173–174

metabolism, 165–167

reducing effect of diabetes, 175

smoking and, 188

X

xanthalesma, 12

Y

yeast infections, 27

blood test for, 53

nutrition and, 115, 120

yoga, 128

Z

Zyban, 192